# Minor Surgery
# at a Glance

This title is also available as an e-book.
For more details, please see
**www.wiley.com/buy/9781118561447**
or scan this QR code:

# Minor Surgery
# at a Glance

**Edited by**

**Helen Mohan**
Department of Surgery
St. Vincent's University Hospital
Dublin, Ireland

**Des Winter**
Department of Surgery
St. Vincent's University Hospital
Dublin, Ireland

WILEY Blackwell

This edition first published 2017 © 2017 by John Wiley and Sons, Ltd.

| Registered office: | John Wiley & Sons, Ltd, The Atrium, Southern Gate, Chichester, West Sussex, PO19 8SQ, UK |
| --- | --- |
| Editorial offices: | 9600 Garsington Road, Oxford, OX4 2DQ, UK |
| | The Atrium, Southern Gate, Chichester, West Sussex, PO19 8SQ, UK |
| | 111 River Street, Hoboken, NJ 07030-5774, USA |

For details of our global editorial offices, for customer services and for information about how to apply for permission to reuse the copyright material in this book please see our website at www.wiley.com/wiley-blackwell

*Library of Congress Cataloging-in-Publication Data*

Names: Mohan, Helen, 1983- editor. | Winter, Desmond, 1969- editor.
Title: Minor surgery at a glance / edited by Helen Mohan, Desmond Winter.
Other titles: At a glance series (Oxford, England)
Description: Chichester, West Sussex : John Wiley & Sons, Ltd,
  2017. | Series: At a glance series | Includes bibliographical references
  and index.
Identifiers: LCCN 2016019921 (print) | LCCN 2016020560 (ebook) | ISBN
  9781118561447 (pbk.) | ISBN 9781118561423 (pdf) | ISBN 9781118561430 (epub)
Subjects: | MESH: Minor Surgical Procedures--methods | Perioperative Care |
  Handbooks
Classification: LCC RD111 (print) | LCC RD111 (ebook) | NLM WO 39 | DDC
  617/.024–dc23
LC record available at https://lccn.loc.gov/2016019921

A catalogue record for this book is available from the British Library.

Wiley also publishes its books in a variety of electronic formats. Some content that appears in print may not be available in electronic books.

Cover image: © Getty/image source

Set in 9.5/11.5 and Minion Pro Regular by Aptara Inc., New Delhi, India
Printed and bound in Singapore by Markono Print Media Pte Ltd

1  2017

# Contents

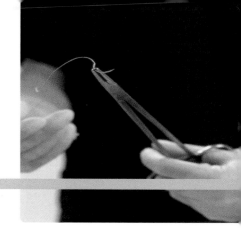

# Contributors

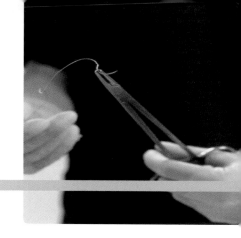

Tan Arulampalam, Chapters 2, 3

Robert Baigrie, Chapter 36

Ishwarya Balasubramanian, Chapters 26, 28

Andrew J Beamish, Chapter 39

Dara Breslin, Chapters 14, 16

Michelle Carey, Chapter 13

Michael Chung, Chapter 24

David J Clark, Chapter 47

Maura Cotter, Chapter 8

Denis Cusack, Chapter 1

Joana Ferrer Fábrega, Chapter 34

Christina Fleming, Chapter 27

Charlotte Florence, Chapter 47

Jessica J Foster, Chapter 39

Greg Fulton, Chapter 37

Olivier Gié, Chapters 9, 21, 22, 23

Amy Godden, Chapter 33

Graeme JK Guthrie, Chapter 30

Hanafiah Harunarashid, Chapter 17

Masakazu Hasegawa, Chapter 38

Anna Heeney, Chapter 37

Paul Horgan, Chapter 30

Steve Hornby, Chapters 13, 46

James Horwood, Chapter 47

Michael Hu, Chapter 43

Jeong Hyun, Chapter 32

Farrah-Hani Imran, Chapter 17

Anand Alister Joseph Ramachandran, Chapter 15

Josep M Grau Junyen, Chapter 34

Genevieve Kelly, Chapters 25–28

Michael Kelly, Chapter 35

Rory Kennelly, Chapter 45

Brian Kirby, Chapters 25–28

Walter Koltun, Chapters 19, 20

Nik Ritza Kosai, Chapter 17

Stavros Koustais, Chapter 31

David Lo, Chapter 18

Michael T Longaker, Chapters 18, 24, 32, 38, 42, 43

Marie-Laure Matthey, Chapters 9, 22

Adrian McArdle, Chapters 18, 24, 32, 38, 42, 43

Frank D McDermott, Chapters 5–7, 33

Keno Mentor, Chapter 36

Helen Mohan, Chapters 4, 23, 25, 31, 37, 41, 48

Nigel Noor, Chapters 2, 3

Maeve O'Connor, Chapter 14

Peter Radford, Chapter 29

Meenakshi Ramphul, Chapter 12

Rish Sehgal, Chapters 19, 20

# Preface

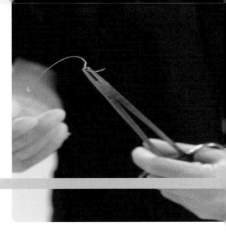

Minor surgery is a generic term encompassing a variety of elective and emergency procedures. The term minor surgery can be misleading, as these operations are far from trivial and serious consequences can arise. Therefore, minor surgery requires due care and consideration. This book provides an overview of minor surgical techniques and common minor surgical procedures.

The first half of the book deals with general principles of minor surgery. These include non-technical factors, for example, how to deal with patients and their families, consent, and technical considerations such as asepsis, wound closure and choice of suture material. The second half of the book covers common minor procedures in both the elective and emergency setting.

This book does not attempt to provide an exhaustive review of minor surgery, but rather to provide a useful starting point to adjunct clinical learning for those embarking on minor surgery, including surgical trainees, GPs and emergency medicine physicians.

*Helen Mohan*
*Des Winter*

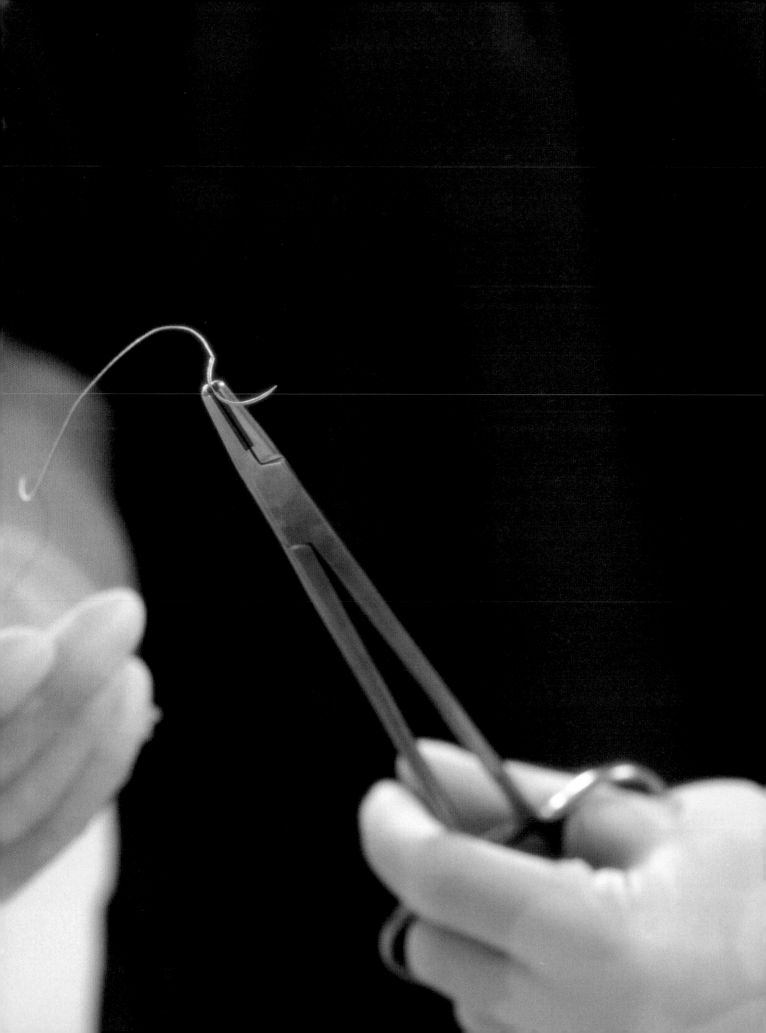

# Avoiding and managing problems: principles of safe surgery

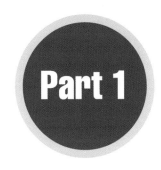

**Part 1**

## Chapters

# 1 Consent

**Box 1.1** Consent and information disclosure: some practical tips on what to do

- Treat the process of obtaining consent from a patient like any other medical procedure for which you should have been fully trained and which you yourself understand
- Proper documentation or recording of the process and disclosed information is a key element whether by brief clinical note or full and signed consent form from the patient
- Have a written aide-memoire of information given to patients for standard procedures in your practice which can be referred to in the event of any subsequent conflict in recollections as to what was said
- Consider providing a written patient information leaflet summarising the main points of the proposed treatment or intervention (including risks and complications)
- Ensure that there is not a mismatch between patient expectation of outcome and what might reasonably be achieved by any proposed intervention
- Ask your patient for a brief replay of what they understand you propose to do and what they believe the expected outcome to be
- Seek medico-legal expert advice in non-standard cases where questions arise

**Box 1.3** Resumé of examples of relevant legislation

### (a) Ireland

***Bunreacht na hÉireann (Constitution of Ireland) Articles 40.1 and 41.1*** – guarantee of personal and family rights

***Non-Fatal Offences Against the Person Act 1997 Section 23*** – consent by a minor over 16 years of age to surgical, medical or dental treatment

***Mental Health Act 2001 Part 4*** – consent to treatment in civil mental health law cases

***Mental Capacity Bill 2008*** – proposed reform of law on capacity, formal and informal decision-making

***Assisted Decision-Making (Capacity) Bill 2013*** – proposed reform of the law relating to persons who require or may require assistance in exercising their decision-making capacity

### (b) England & Wales, Northern Ireland and Scotland

***Family Law Reform Act 1969; Age of Majority Act 1969 (Northern Ireland); Age of Legal Capacity (Scotland) Act 1991; and Adults with Incapacity (Scotland) Act 2000*** – competence and capacity of children and adults generally

***Mental Capacity Act 2005*** – relating to decision making where persons lack capacity

***Mental Health Care and Treatment (Scotland) Act 2003*** – providing for the treatment of people if they have a mental disorder

**Box 1.2** Summary of judgements from some landmark court cases

### (a) Examples of Irish court decisions

***Re A Ward of Court (withholding medical treatment)*** *(No. 2) (1996) 2 IR 79* – the Supreme Court considered in detail the best interests approach in circumstances where the patient in a near persistent vegetative state was unable to give consent or refusal herself.

***Geoghegan v Harris*** *(2000) 3 IR 536* – in a dental negligence case, the High Court considered the duty of a doctor to disclose on the standard principles of medical negligence and what to disclose on the reasonable patient test.

***North Western Health Board v H W and C W*** *(2001) 3 IR 622* – the Supreme Court set out the balance to be achieved between the child's rights and that of the parents in the circumstances of the parents' considered refusal to permit a heel-prick PKU test to be performed.

***Fitzpatrick v White*** *(2007) IESC 51* – the Supreme Court analysed the practicalities of obtaining informed consent in good time prior to elective day surgery in ophthamology.

***Fitzpatrick and Ryan v FK and Attorney General*** *(2008) IEHC 104* – the High Court considered the parameters of capacity in an adult patient refusing a life-saving blood transfusion.

### (b) Examples of other common law decisions

***Gillick v West Norfolk and Wisbech Area Health Authority*** *(1985) 3 All ER 402 (HL)* – the House of Lords ruled that a child under the age of sixteen may have the necessary competence for capacity for decision making in certain circumstances.

***Rogers v Whitaker*** *(1992) 175 CLR 479* – the Australian Courts ruled that the risk of total blindness from an ophthalmological procedure, although very small, was material to the patient's decision considering her particular clinical circumstances and that it was negligent not to advise her of that risk.

***Chester v Afshar*** *(2004) UKHL 41* – the House of Lords held in a discectomy case that doctors must warn patients about all material risks (in this case, 'a small but unavoidable risk that the proposed operation, however expertly performed' might lead to cauda equina syndrome) and that patients be given time to consider their options before deciding whether or not to undergo the treatment or explore other options.

***Foo Fio Na v Soo Fook Mun & Assunta Hospital*** *(2007) 1MLJ 593* – the Malaysian Federal Court held in a case related to the surgical treatment of the plaintiff following a motor vehicle accident suffered by her in July 1982 resulting in cervical vertebra dislocation that the *Rogers v Whitaker* test applied to the duty to disclose information to patients.

***Montgomery v Lanarkshire Health Board*** *(2015) UKSC 11* – the UK Supreme Court moved decisively from the `reasonable doctor' test (Bolam and Sidaway cases) to the `reasonable patient' test in a case of cerebral palsy outcome where consent for vaginal delivery was sought without explanation of caesarian section option.

**Box 1.4** Examples of helpful professional advisory publications

| (a) Ireland | (b) United Kingdom and other common law jurisdictions |
|---|---|
| ***Guide to Professional Conduct and Ethics for Registered Medical Practitioners, Chapter 3 and Appendix C*** *(8th Edition, 2016).* Medical Council of Ireland | ***Consent: patients and doctors making decisions together*** *(2008).* General Medical Council |
| ***Good Medical Practice in Seeking Informed Consent to Treatment*** *(2008).* Medical Council of Ireland | ***Consent tool kit*** *(2008).* British Medical Association<br>***Consent Guideline for Treatment of Patients by Registered Medical Practitioners*** *(2013).* Malaysian Medical Council |
| ***Operational Procedures for Research Ethics Committees: Guidance 2004.*** Irish Council for Bioethics | ***Good Medical Practice: a Code of Conduct for Doctors in Australia*** *(2014).* Medical Board of Australia |

*Minor Surgery at a Glance*, First Edition. Edited by Helen Mohan and Desmond Winter. © 2017 John Wiley & Sons, Ltd. Published 2017 by John Wiley & Sons, Ltd.

# The nature of consent

This medico-legal summary is based on current laws in Common Law jurisdictions (those which have their roots in the English legal system). The principles are, however, applicable to medical practice across other legal systems.

A doctor is obliged to obtain a patient's prior agreement to any proposed treatment, intervention or procedure. This respects the patient's right to be involved in their healthcare decisions. Consent may be implied from the conduct of the patient or circumstances of the consultation. But where there is an intervention or procedure with potential side effects or adverse outcome, then express consent, either verbal or written, must be obtained. Allegations of clinical negligence in cases of adverse or unexpected outcome now frequently include an allegation of failure to obtain proper informed consent in addition to allegations of negligent performance standard.

## The three core elements of consent

**(i)** Competence or capacity: A person is deemed to have capacity if they have the ability to understand the information given by the doctor, to weigh it up and to make a decision as to whether to accept or refuse the proposed treatment or procedure. The person must also be able to communicate this decision clearly. Particular care is required for a child under the age of legal consent (commonly 16 years); or where there is doubt about the mental health or intellectual ability of the patient; or if there is a physical difficulty impeding clear communication. In all of these circumstances, detailed consideration must be given to assessing capacity and there may be a need for the doctor to consult a medico-legal advisor.
**(ii)** Voluntariness: The doctor must also be satisfied that the patient is giving consent voluntarily and is not under any duress, coercion or undue pressure from any other person to either accept or refuse the proposed treatment or intervention.
**(iii)** Information disclosure: Providing sufficient information to the patient is a critical element of obtaining valid consent and the emphasis has shifted onto this element in modern clinical practice and medical law. It is also the most difficult element to define medico-legally.

The patient should be given information regarding:
**1** Their condition, illness or disease
**2** The nature, scope and significance of any proposed treatment or intervention
**3** The aims and expected outcome
**4** Any discomfort, common side effect or risks of the procedure
**5** Any alternative or choices of treatment.

The patient must also be told that they are free to refuse treatment or to withdraw their consent at any time prior to the treatment.

# How detailed should information be?

Different levels of detail are required to be given depending on the nature of the intervention. In all cases, the standard is what a reasonable person would expect to be told in order to make a fully informed decision. The standard level of information given to the patient must include an explanation of any frequent minor risks and of major risks (even if infrequent), which are sometimes referred to as 'material risks'. In the case of medical necessity for the procedure there is a general and approved practice not to disclose minimal risks that might cause unnecessary anxiety and stress or might deter the patient from undergoing necessary treatment, but this must be the exception rather than the rule. When the procedure is not a medical necessity (sometimes called 'elective'), the required standard of information provision is higher and tends towards full disclosure. Disclosure must also include direct and full response to specific questions raised by the patient about the procedure, including any complications. It is the substance of the disclosure that is critical to the validity of the consent rather than the mere formulaic existence of a written and signed consent form.

# What is material risk?

The legal analysis of the meaning of material risk by the Courts has changed in recent times. The question of risk is no longer solely determined by the standards of the medical profession but is judged by the significance a reasonable patient would attach to the risk of the proposed treatment or intervention. What constitutes material risk involves consideration of both the severity of the potential consequences and the statistical frequency of the risk.

# The adult patient

A competent adult patient must make the decision about a treatment or intervention themselves. No one else is entitled to make that decision for them. If not competent, then other persons may be in a position to contribute to such a decision using a combination of tests of substituted judgment (as if standing in the shoes of the patient) and 'best interests' of the patient. In the event of a dispute between next-of-kin and/or health carers over such a decision, the Courts may ultimately be asked to make the decision.

# The child patient

In the majority of Common Law jurisdictions, statute laws are in place by which a child under 18 years but who is 16 years or over is considered legally competent to give consent to medical, surgical or dental treatment. However, doctors should be familiar with local, national or state legal provisions that provide for varied age thresholds (e.g. from 14 to 18 years). The parents or legal guardians of a child under the relevant legal age are considered entitled to give consent on behalf of the child. A mature child under that age may in certain defined circumstances be considered competent. The Courts will have the ultimate decision where a dispute arises or where the refusal of treatment is considered potentially detrimental to the child.

# The patient with cognitive impairment or intellectual disability

Great care must be taken in circumstances where the capacity of the adult patient to make decisions is in doubt. In cases of dispute or in the absence of clear agreement or legal authority, the Courts will be the ultimate decision maker.

# Seeking medico-legal advice

When a doctor is faced with a situation where there is doubt about the validity of the consent of the patient or where there is disagreement about treatment or intervention when a patient is not considered competent to make such a decision, the doctor is advised to seek immediate expert medico-legal advice from their medical indemnity organisation. The only exception in this scenario is in circumstances of medical emergency where there is an immediate danger to the health or well-being of the patient, when the doctor may have to act in the patient's best clinical interest. Doctors should also seek such expert advice if in doubt in any specific consent situation.

# 2 Physical environment

**Table 2.1** Free-standing versus hospital-integrated units for minor surgery

| | Advantages | Disadvantages |
|---|---|---|
| **Free-standing** | • Patient travelling distances and times are minimised<br>• More efficient use of resources, maximising throughput of selected procedures and minimising the cost per patient | • Lack of overnight facilities constrains both patient eligibility and case mix<br>• If a patient is unable to be safely discharged when the free-standing unit closes in the evening, they require ambulance transfer to the main hospital<br>• Lack of backup facilities in emergencies |
| **Hospital integrated units** | • Availability of additional resources as required<br>• Availability of short-stay beds allows treatment to be performed on less surgically fit patients and for more complex operations | • Further distances for patients to travel<br>• More expensive to operate than community-based services<br>• Subject to external hospital pressures such as bed shortages and staffing issues leading to list cancellations |

*Minor Surgery at a Glance,* First Edition. Edited by Helen Mohan and Desmond Winter. © 2017 John Wiley & Sons, Ltd. Published 2017 by John Wiley & Sons, Ltd.

## Suitable settings for minor surgery

Minor surgery should ideally be conducted in an environment specifically designed for that purpose. Minor surgery services may be separated from the inpatient hospital environment in favour of hospital-integrated units or community-based free-standing units (often referred to as Treatment Centres or Ambulatory Care and Diagnostic Centres (ACADs) in the UK). There are several advantages and disadvantages to hospital-based versus community-based units (Table 2.1). Patient selection is key if using a community-based unit, as the same backup is not present as in the hospital environment.

## Facilities required

Minor surgery facilities can be configured in a number of ways but generally require a day ward or waiting area to receive patients, operating theatres or procedure rooms and a recovery area for rehabilitation. In the hospital setting, anaesthetic rooms are often also used. Modernisation of medical practice has led to the replacement of beds in favour of trolleys and chairs to reduce space requirements and also to promote earlier mobilisation to aid recovery.

For general practitioners setting up a minor operating facility, it is important to be aware of health and safety legislation and to ensure that sterilisation of equipment, sharps disposal and use of chemicals such as liquid nitrogen complies with relevant health and safety legislation.

## What factors are important to the layout of the operating theatre complex?

The physical layout of the operating suite can be variable; however, recognition of the importance of reducing contamination to reduce wound infection has led to the delineation of clean, hazardous and contaminated areas as seen here.

### Unrestricted – contaminated

These include the patient receiving area, dressing rooms, lounges and office.

### Semi-restricted – hazardous

These include hallways, instrument and supply processing area, storage areas and utility rooms.

### Restricted – clean

These include the operating theatre, scrub sink areas and sterile supply rooms.

## What are the design and equipment requirements for a minor surgery-operating suite?

### Cleanliness

The surgery-operating suite must be spacious to allow scrubbed personnel to move around non-sterile equipment without contamination. In addition, it must be easy to clean – uncluttered and simple so that dust is not trapped in areas that would be difficult to clean. Surfaces must be durable and easy to clean to reduce contamination.

### Ventilation

Guidelines for the design of new operating theatre facilities advocate positive pressure ventilation of 25 exchanges per hour of filtered air. Windows should not be opened. However, a facility with natural ventilation is acceptable for most minor surgical procedures. If using natural ventilation, windows can be opened but only if they have an adequate fly screen. Humidity is controlled to 50–53% to achieve minimal static and reduce microbial growth. Temperature is maintained at 20–24 °C.

### Lighting and equipment

It is important to have appropriate lighting – both in terms of overhead room lights and surgical spotlights for the operative site. The operating table should be adjustable for height, degree of tilt in all directions, orientation in the room, articular breaks and length.

### Safety

It is important to have a telephone to contact outside assistance. Emergency numbers should be clearly displayed.

Anaesthesia equipment and monitoring as appropriate to the surgery must be present and in good condition. Anaesthetic machines must be checked at the start of every case.

Fire safety is crucial and the theatre should be designed in keeping with fire regulations.

### Further reading

Humphreys H, Coia JE, Stacey A, et al. Guidelines on the facilities required for minor surgical procedures and minimal access intervention. *Journal of Hospital Infection* 2012; 80: 103–109.

# 3 Set-up

**Figure 3.1** Patient positioning in surgery

| Position | Exposure | Risks |
|---|---|---|
| **Supine** | Abdomen, face, neck chest, shoulder | • Ulnar nerve<br>• Peroneal nerve |
| **Prone** | Posterior torso, buttocks | • Difficult anaesthesia<br>• Airway tube dislodgment<br>• Pressure damage to face/eyes |
| **Trendelenburg** | Pelvic organs | • Stress on diaphragm leading to breathing restriction<br>• Slide from table<br>• Shoulder rests can lead to brachial plexus injury |
| **Reverse trendelenburg** | Face, neck | • Slide from table |
| **Kraske** (jackknife) | Anorectum | • Pressure on male genitals |
| **Lithotomy** | Vagina, perineum, rectum | • Raise legs slowly to avoid BP changes<br>• Avoid hip dislocation<br>• Avoid fingers trapped in table hinges<br>• Peroneal nerve injury |
| **Fowler** (sitting) | Face, neck, mouth | |
| **Sims** (lateral) | Flank, kidney, ureters, lung | • Pressure to bony prominences on underside of patient |

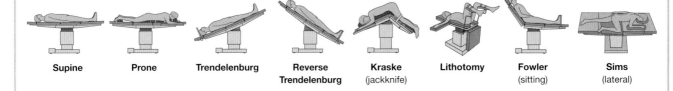

| Supine | Prone | Trendelenburg | Reverse Trendelenburg | Kraske (jackknife) | Lithotomy | Fowler (sitting) | Sims (lateral) |

**Figure 3.2** Set-up of operating room

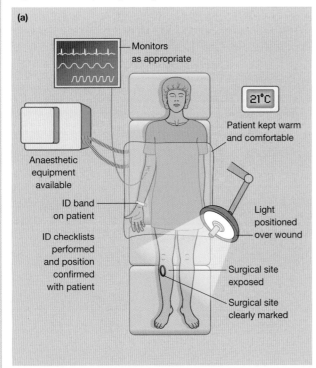

(a)
- Monitors as appropriate
- 21°C
- Patient kept warm and comfortable
- Anaesthetic equipment available
- ID band on patient
- ID checklists performed and position confirmed with patient
- Light positioned over wound
- Surgical site exposed
- Surgical site clearly marked

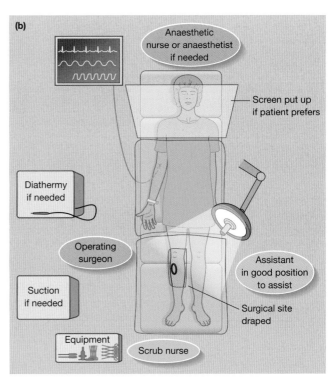

(b)
- Anaesthetic nurse or anaesthetist if needed
- Screen put up if patient prefers
- Diathermy if needed
- Operating surgeon
- Suction if needed
- Equipment
- Scrub nurse
- Assistant in good position to assist
- Surgical site draped

*Minor Surgery at a Glance,* First Edition. Edited by Helen Mohan and Desmond Winter. © 2017 John Wiley & Sons, Ltd. Published 2017 by John Wiley & Sons, Ltd.

# Patient positioning

## Why is patient positioning important?

Operating surgeons have the ethical responsibility of treating their patients with the principle of non-maleficence. The anaesthetised patient loses their ability to communicate pain and pressure to the surgical team, and therefore it is now *your* responsibility to ensure the patient is positioned safely (Figure 3.1). The American Society of Anaesthesiologists (ASA) provides useful guidelines on positioning intraoperatively.

## What are the goals of patient positioning?

The goal of the surgical position is to provide optimal exposure of the surgical site that causes the least physiological compromise of the patient, while also protecting the skin and joints. For conscious patients, it is also important to consider comfortable positioning that can be sustained for the duration of the operation without the need to alter position, which may risk destabilisation of the operation site. Other considerations include allowing access for the administration of IV fluids and anaesthetic agents, and access to the patient for surgical/radiological equipment (Figure 3.2).

## Lighting

It is generally easier to position lights yourself prior to draping and to ensure that there is someone available to move the light during the procedure if needed, and that you have a sterile light handle if you need to adjust the light quickly. In general, light should come from behind and over the shoulder of the operating surgeon. Make sure that you maintain your posture and you are not bending into the wound. This will maintain your own back health and prevent you impeding the light and being an infection hazard.

## Equipment

Ideally, any anticipated special equipment, such as diathermy, should be set up or at least be readily available at the start of the procedure. Also consider whether the patient is warm enough – a Bair Hugger™ or similar device may be needed – and whether the patient wishes to have a screen so that they cannot see the operation.

## Assistance

Assistants are important for providing adequate access in an operation. If you are embarking on a difficult or challenging case, a skilled assistant can make a huge difference to the ease of the procedure overall. If you have an inexperienced assistant, make sure that you brief them at the start of the case on what the plan is and on what you will likely need them to do. Keep instructions clear and succinct during the procedure and check in regularly that the assistant understands and is happy with what they are doing.

# Surgical safety

## Skin marking

Skin marking of the surgical site is important to ensure correct site surgery on the correct patient. Marking the site should be carried out at the time of confirmation of consent. Involvement of the patient in the skin marking process is important in ensuring correct site surgery. Therefore, marking should be carried out before the patient has received any premedication sedation. Before marking the site, confirm that it is the correct site in the notes, the relevant imaging, the consent and with the patient. The mark should be close to the proposed incision site and unambiguous, for example a line rather than a cross. Institutional guidelines may exist to guide the preferred marking method.

Marks should be made using a permanent non-water-soluble marker pointing to the surgical site. In theatre, additional skin marking may be undertaken to demonstrate the precise proposed incision site. This should be undertaken prior to infiltration of local anaesthetic which may distort tissue planes.

## Time out

The WHO surgical safety checklist is used to improve patient safety by confirming the surgical site and identifying any allergies or surgical or anaesthetic concerns.

# Preparation of the surgical site

## Hair removal

Hair removal from incision sites is controversial. In general, hair should only be removed when necessary. Hair removal should be performed in theatre. A clipper rather than a razor should be used for hair removal.

## Skin preparation

Surgical skin preparation options include povidone-iodine or chlorhexidine with or without ethanol. For further details on the selection of the agent see Chapter 5 Infection control and prevention. Drapes made of linen (muslin) or paper (non-woven) are then placed over the patient to leave only the surgical site exposed.

### Further reading

American Society of Anesthesiologists Task Force on Prevention of Perioperative Peripheral Neuropathies. Practice advisory for the prevention of perioperative peripheral neuropathies: an updated report by the American Society of Anesthesiologists Task Force on prevention of perioperative peripheral neuropathies. *Anesthesiology* 2011; 114(4): 741–754.

http://www.has-sante.fr/portail/upload/docs/application/pdf/2013-05/guide_to_surgical_site_marking.pdf (accessed 20 May 2016).

# 4 Instruments

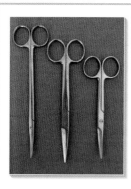

**Figure 4.1**
From left to right:
Metzenbaum,
Straight Mayo
and Curved
Mayo scissors

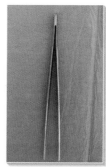

**Figure 4.2**   DeBakey forceps

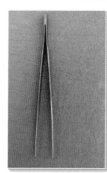

**Figure 4.3**   Toothed forceps

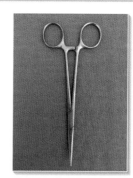

**Figure 4.4**
Artery forceps/clip/
haemostat

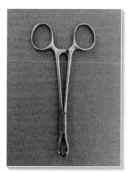

**Figure 4.5**
Lane's tissue holding
forceps

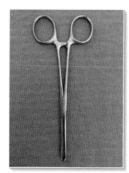

**Figure 4.6**   Allis tissue holding forceps

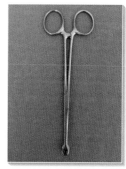

**Figure 4.7**   Babcock's
tissue holding forceps

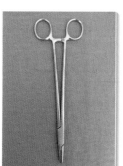

**Figure 4.8**   Needle holder

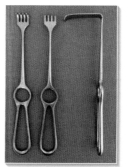

**Figure 4.9**
left: Rake retractors
right: Langenbeck retractor

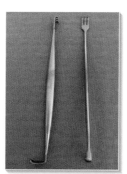

**Figure 4.10**   Cat's paws retractors

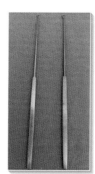

**Figure 4.11**   Skin hooks

*Minor Surgery at a Glance*, First Edition. Edited by Helen Mohan and Desmond Winter. © 2017 John Wiley & Sons, Ltd. Published 2017 by John Wiley & Sons, Ltd.

Appropriate knowledge of instruments is essential for performing minor surgery. Minor surgery, like all surgery, often relies on good retraction to show the tissue planes for dissection with minimal blood loss and in good anatomical planes. Instruments often have multiple names and terminology can vary in different parts of the world and from institution to institution, so familiarise yourself with local instrument names whenever you move institution.

## Scissors

There are several types of scissors used in minor operations (Figure 4.1). There are the Metzenbaum dissecting scissors, commonly called 'Metz' scissors. These have a delicate fine tip. The other common scissors are straight and curved Mayo scissors. A curved Mayo scissors may be used to cut tough tissues like fascia. Cutting sutures with the fine tip of the Metzenbaum can cause damage to the scissors and Mayo scissors should be used instead.

## Grasping forceps

There are several types of forceps used for grasping tissues. These include toothed, non-toothed, DeBakey and Russian forceps (Figures 4.2 and 4.3).

In general, toothed forceps are used for the skin and to hold a bleeder for diathermy. Non-toothed or DeBakey forceps are used for more delicate tissue handling. Smaller forceps – e.g. Adson forceps – are useful for closing the skin and for delicate work.

## Clips

Artery forceps/clip (or haemostat) or the smaller mosquito forceps may be used to occlude vessels (Figure 4.4).

## Tissue holders

There are a number of instruments used to grasp tissues. These include Lane's (Figure 4.5), Kocher's, Allis (Figure 4.6) and Babcock's (Figure 4.7) tissue holding forceps. Care must be taken as these instruments can cause damage to tissue and should be avoided on delicate or damaged tissue.

## Needle holder

A needle holder can vary in size and heaviness depending on the tissue being sutured. In general, heavy needle holders are used for thick tissue and lighter needle holders are used for delicate work (Figure 4.8). A long needle holder should be used for suturing deep in a cavity, while a shorter needle holder is appropriate for surface tissues. In general, the length of the needle holder and the forceps should be equal.

## Retractors

Much successful surgery depends on adequate retraction. There are several retractors that are useful in minor surgery. Langenbeck retractors generally come in small, medium and large sizes (Figure 4.9).

For smaller and more delicate work, smaller retractors like cat's paws (Figure 4.10) or skin hooks (Figure 4.11) can be useful.

# 5 Infection control and prevention

**Figure 5.1** Surgical site infection bundle

Maintain normothermia

Appropriate antibiotic prophylaxis (started and finished promptly)

**Surgical site infection bundle**

Maintain glucose levels

Appropriate hair removal

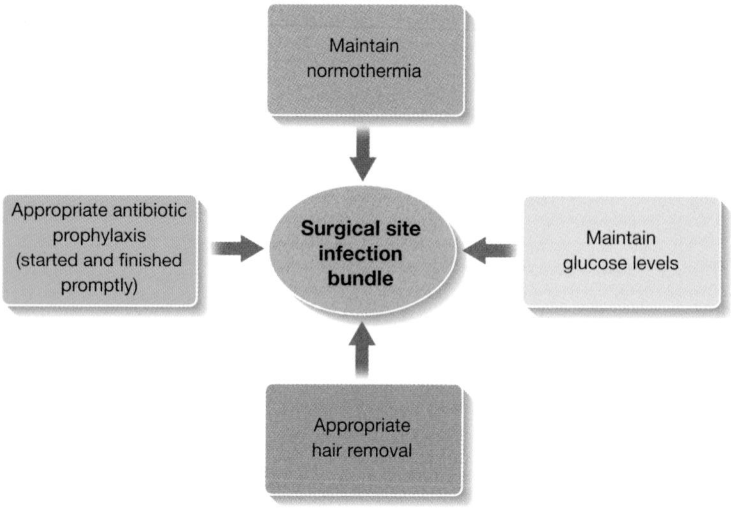

**Figure 5.2 Sterilisation techniques**

**Radiation**
Ionising (e.g. gamma)
Non ionising (e.g. ultraviolet)

**Sterilisation techniques**

**Heat**
(e.g. steam autoclave 121°C for 15 mins)

**Chemical**
(e.g. ethylene oxide, bleach, glutaraldehyde)

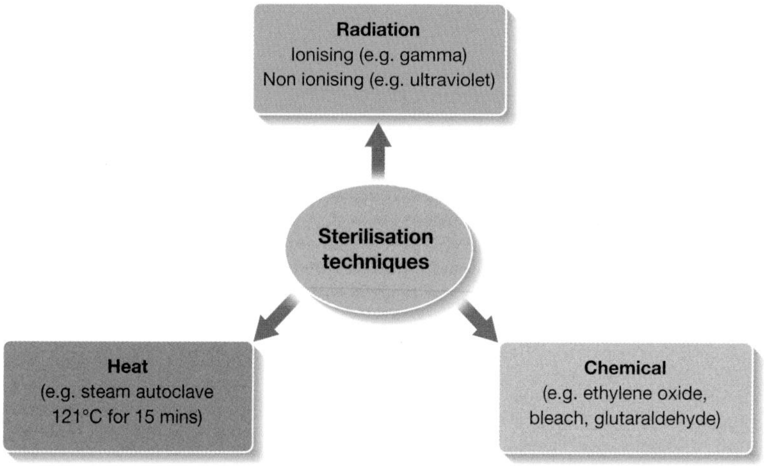

**Figure 5.3** Characteristics of two commonly used skin preparation solutions; povidone iodine and chlorhexidine

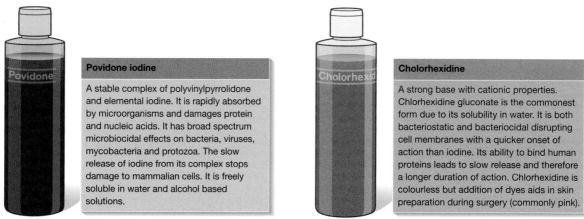

**Povidone iodine**

A stable complex of polyvinylpyrrolidone and elemental iodine. It is rapidly absorbed by microorganisms and damages protein and nucleic acids. It has broad spectrum microbiocidal effects on bacteria, viruses, mycobacteria and protozoa. The slow release of iodine from its complex stops damage to mammalian cells. It is freely soluble in water and alcohol based solutions.

**Cholorhexidine**

A strong base with cationic properties. Chlorhexidine gluconate is the commonest form due to its solubility in water. It is both bacteriostatic and bacteriocidal disrupting cell membranes with a quicker onset of action than iodine. Its ability to bind human proteins leads to slow release and therefore a longer duration of action. Chlorhexidine is colourless but addition of dyes aids in skin preparation during surgery (commonly pink).

*Minor Surgery at a Glance,* First Edition. Edited by Helen Mohan and Desmond Winter. © 2017 John Wiley & Sons, Ltd. Published 2017 by John Wiley & Sons, Ltd.

# Infection prevention

Semmelweiss first demonstrated that use of chlorinated lime solutions reduced puerperal sepsis in 1847. Modern surgery demands rigorous infection control practices to reduce the serious morbidity associated with post-operative infections. Endogenous infection is caused by organisms present on the patient on admission, while cross-infection is caused by organisms acquired during the admission from other patients or staff.

## Types of pathogens

Pathogens can be classified into conventional, conditional and opportunistic. Conventional pathogens cause disease in healthy subjects in the absence of pre-existing immunity (e.g. *Staphylococcus*, tuberculosis, and hepatitis viruses). Conditional pathogens – such as *Pseudomonas aeruginosa* and *Candida* spp. – cause disease in patients with reduced immunity (e.g. newborns) and also if directly implanted into a sterile area (e.g. following surgery). Opportunistic pathogens – such as *Pneumocystis carinii* – only cause disease in patients who are severely immunocompromised.

## Routes of transmission

**Direct:** Transmission of infection from another patient, health-care worker or visitor.

**Indirect:** Transmission of an infection from an object or surface that an infected patient has previously interacted with.

**Air:** Transmission of infectious organisms into the air for example, by coughing and sneezing.

**Vector:** Transmission of infection via, for example, insects or parasites.

# Minor surgery and infection

Several care bundles have been proposed to reduce the incidence of surgical site infection (SSI) by attention to perioperative detail (Figure 5.1).

## Preoperative phase

Advise patients to shower/bathe with normal soap on the day prior or day of surgery. Previous studies have shown that either normal soap or chlorhexidine washing before an operation reduces risk of infection.

**Hair removal:** Can cause tissue damage and release bacterial organisms. Therefore, hair should not be removed unless required for the procedure. If needed, remove hair with electrical clippers with a single use head just prior to the procedure.

**Antibiotics:** Should not be routinely used for most minor surgical procedures. They are usually reserved for procedures involving the use of prostheses/implants or clean contaminated/contaminated procedures. If required, adequate time should be allowed for the antibiotic to reach the desired plasma concentration before 'knife to skin'.

## Operative phase

**Hand decontamination:** Hands and nails should be washed thoroughly with antiseptic solution prior to operating. Soap and water remove contaminants and most microbial organisms but antiseptic solution is required to destroy resistant organisms and those deep in hair follicles. In between operative cases alcohol solution or antiseptic solution should be used. Apply a sterile gown using an aseptic technique.

Prepare operative field with suitable antiseptic solution, the most commonly used are aqueous or alcohol based iodine and chlorhexidine (Figure 5.3). Recent evidence supports alcohol-based chlorhexidine compared to iodine. Caution must be exercised with alcohol based solutions particularly in areas where the solution can pool as it poses a fire risk with diathermy.

## Sterilising Instruments

It is important to distinguish disinfection that destroys specific pathogenic organisms compared with sterilisation that destroys all organisms including resistant spores. Sterilisation can be achieved by multiple means. The most commonly employed include high temperature (e.g. steam autoclave), chemical (e.g. ethylene oxide) and radiation (e.g. gamma) (Figure 5.2).

**Wound closure:** Aim to close parallel to Langer's lines, ensure that the wound is tension free (you may need to undermine the skin edges) and use suitable suture material. There is no evidence demonstrating an advantage between absorbable and non-absorbable sutures in terms of SSI.

Cover the wound with a dressing at the end of the procedure for 48 hours.

## Post-operative phase

Patients may shower after 48 hours.

Inform patients of potential signs of infection – worsening pain, spreading redness/cellulitis, pyrexia, pus – and that they should seek medical advice if concerned.

Take microbiological swabs and treat suspected infection with antibiotics to treat likely causative organisms, taking into consideration local microbial patterns.

Infection control in hospitals involves many different components such as to reduce spread, for example isolating the infection by using individual patient rooms and barrier nursing. It must be assumed that all clinical areas are potential sources of infection and therefore 'standard' precautions are undertaken in all hospitals (i.e. hand washing, gloves, gowns and eye protection) if there is a risk of bodily fluids splashing. Hospitals should have adequate facilities to clean linen and to sterilise/disinfect instruments, and policies to reduce the risk of accidental blood-borne pathogen inoculation (e.g. sharps bins, safe needles and cannulae).

### Further reading

Carrick MM, Miller HJ, Awad SS, et al. Chlorhexidine-alcohol versus povidone-iodine for surgical-site antisepsis. *New England Journal of Medicine* 2010; 362(1): 18-26. doi: 10.1056/NEJMoa0810988.

Darouiche RO, Wall MJ Jr, Itani KM, et al. Implementation of a bundle of care to reduce surgical site infections in patients undergoing vascular surgery. *PLoS One* 2013: 8(8): e71566.

Tanner J, Norrie P, Melen K. Preoperative hair removal to reduce surgical site infection. *Cochrane Database Systematic Review* 2011 Nov 9;(11):CD004122.

# 6 Human factors

**Table 6.1** Surgical safety checklist. Reproduced with permission of WHO.

## SURGICAL SAFETY CHECKLIST (FIRST EDITION)

Before induction of anaesthesia ▶▶▶▶▶▶▶▶ Before skin incision ▶▶▶▶▶▶▶▶▶▶▶▶ Before patient leaves operating room

### SIGN IN

☐ PATIENT HAS CONFIRMED
- IDENTITY
- SITE
- PROCEDURE
- CONSENT

☐ SITE MARKED/NOT APPLICABLE

☐ ANAESTHESIA SAFETY CHECK COMPLETED

☐ PULSE OXIMETER ON PATIENT AND FUNCTIONING

DOES PATIENT HAVE A:

KNOWN ALLERGY?
☐ NO
☐ YES

DIFFICULT AIRWAY/ASPIRATION RISK?
☐ NO
☐ YES, AND EQUIPMENT/ASSISTANCE AVAILABLE

RISK OF >500ML BLOOD LOSS
(7ML/KG IN CHILDREN)?
☐ NO
☐ YES, AND ADEQUATE INTRAVENOUS ACCESS AND FLUIDS PLANNED

### TIME OUT

☐ CONFIRM ALL TEAM MEMBERS HAVE INTRODUCED THEMSELVES BY NAME AND ROLE

☐ SURGEON, ANAESTHESIA PROFESSIONAL AND NURSE VERBALLY CONFIRM
- PATIENT
- SITE
- PROCEDURE

ANTICIPATED CRITICAL EVENTS

☐ SURGEON REVIEWS: WHAT ARE THE CRITICAL OR UNEXPECTED STEPS, OPERATIVE DURATION, ANTICIPATED BLOOD LOSS?

☐ ANAESTHESIA TEAM REVIEWS : ARE THERE ANY PATIENT-SPECIFIC CONCERNS?

☐ NURSING TEAM REVIEWS: HAS STERILITY (INCLUDING INDICATOR RESULTS) BEEN CONFIRMED? ARE THERE EQUIPMENT ISSUES OR ANY CONCERNS?

HAS ANTIBIOTIC PROPHYLAXIS BEEN GIVEN WITHIN THE LAST 60 MINUTES?
☐ YES
☐ NOT APPLICABLE

IS ESSENTIAL IMAGING DISPLAYED?
☐ YES
☐ NOT APPLICABLE

### SIGN OUT

NURSE VERBALLY CONFIRMS WITH THE TEAM:

☐ THE NAME OF THE PROCEDURE RECORDED

☐ THAT INSTRUMENT, SPONGE AND NEEDLE COUNTS ARE CORRECT (OR NOT APPLICABLE)

☐ HOW THE SPECIMEN IS LABELLED (INCLUDING PATIENT NAME)

☐ WHETHER THERE ARE ANY EQUIPMENT PROBLEMS TO BE ADDRESSED

☐ SURGEON, ANAESTHESIA PROFESSIONAL AND NURSE REVIEW THE KEY CONCERNS FOR RECOVERY AND MANAGEMENT OF THIS PATIENT

THIS CHECKLIST IS NOT INTENDED TO BE COMPREHENSIVE. ADDITIONS AND MODIFICATIONS TO FIT LOCAL PRACTICE ARE ENCOURAGED.

**Figure 6.1** Positive safety culture

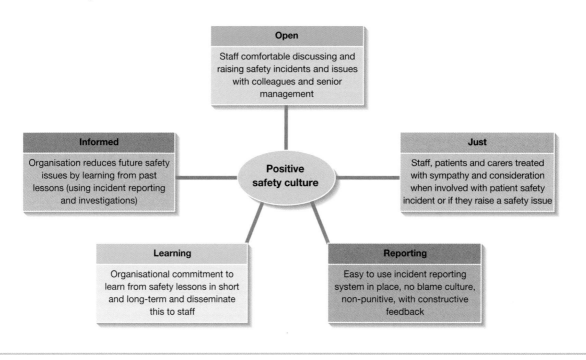

**Open**
Staff comfortable discussing and raising safety incidents and issues with colleagues and senior management

**Informed**
Organisation reduces future safety issues by learning from past lessons (using incident reporting and investigations)

**Positive safety culture**

**Just**
Staff, patients and carers treated with sympathy and consideration when involved with patient safety incident or if they raise a safety issue

**Learning**
Organisational commitment to learn from safety lessons in short and long-term and disseminate this to staff

**Reporting**
Easy to use incident reporting system in place, no blame culture, non-punitive, with constructive feedback

*Minor Surgery at a Glance*, First Edition. Edited by Helen Mohan and Desmond Winter. © 2017 John Wiley & Sons, Ltd. Published 2017 by John Wiley & Sons, Ltd.

# What are human factors?

Poor communication is a major contributing factor in over half of all incidents of harm in hospitals. Operations are complex with multiple factors that must be carefully managed to ensure that the patient receives the correct treatment in a timely and safe manner whilst maintaining dignity. Surgical training in many jurisdictions now includes training in human factors as part of the curriculum, covering a variety of non-technical skills such as communication skills, error, patient safety, consent and interaction with colleagues, and using tools such as simulation. Improving systems to reduce surgical error include checklist initiatives to improve patient safety.

# Safe surgery initiatives

## World Health Organisation (WHO) checklist

The WHO established the 'safe surgery saves lives' initiative to improve surgical outcomes and avoid potential minor and catastrophic errors. They launched the 'surgical safety checklist', which has three components: a 'sign in', 'time out' and 'sign out'. This checklist can be applied globally and the template can be adapted to suit local practices (Table 6.1). The checklist aims to improve outcomes and reduce the incidence of 'never events' in surgery. 'Never events' are errors that 'should never occur', such as wrong patient or wrong site surgery. However, despite this, these events still occur with alarming regularity and every effort to improve patient safety by addressing human factors is necessary. Patient safety organisations have adopted the WHO approach; for example, the National Patient Safety Agency (NPSA) in the UK, have published a 'how to guide' on five steps to safer surgery using adapted WHO guidelines.

These five steps are: (1) briefing, (2) sign in, (3) time out, (4) sign out and (5) debriefing.

**1** Briefing: improves information exchange and the 'smooth' running of a theatre list: introduce names and roles; define objectives; identify major steps; check critical treatment and equipment; ask 'What if?'; check understanding by read back.

**2** Sign in: this occurs in the anaesthetic room and involves confirming that you have the correct patient, correct consent/operation and laterality, drug allergies, potential for haemorrhage and that anaesthetic equipment is working correctly.

**3** Time out: occurs in theatre with all members of the team present to introduce themselves and their role. The patient, site and operation are confirmed. Surgeon reviews the critical steps and equipment for the procedure. Anaesthetist reviews any patient specific concerns. Theatre staff confirm sterility and availability of equipment. Finally, the need for antibiotic and thromboprophylaxis is reviewed.

**4** Sign out: involves the nursing staff confirming the procedure, swab/equipment count and ensuring specimens are labelled. Surgeon, anaesthetist and nursing staff highlight any important factors for the recovery and post-operative management of the patient.

**5** Debriefing: 'How did we feel?', 'What went well?', 'What went not so well?', 'What should we do next time?', 'How did we do?'. Team leader sums up at the end of the debrief to reiterate what has been discussed and to check that there is a shared understanding in the team.

## Improving the working environment

There are seven areas that can be addressed to improve patient care and the working environment. These include:

**1** Cognition and workload: self-awareness of the stressors that we bring to the workplace, and training to deal with this in emergency situations, e.g. simulation, team training.

**2** Distraction avoidance.

**3** Attention to the physical environment (e.g. lighting)

**4** Awareness of the need for rest and not attempting skills outside your capability.

**5** Devices/product design: awareness of heterogeneity in product design from different companies.

**6** Teamwork: good communication (Situation–Background–Assessment–Response [SBAR]) (de)briefing, surgical checklists.

**7** Process design: simplifying steps in complex tasks to minimise mistakes.

*(Adapted from implementing human factors in healthcare, https://www.england.nhs.uk/wp-content/uploads/2013/11/nqb-hum-fact-concord.pdf)*

# Asking for help

It is important to recognise your limitations and to realise when to call for help. Prior to any procedure, anticipate what help may be needed (e.g. a senior colleague, an anaesthetist) and ensure that they will be available if required. Make sure theatre staff know how to call for help in the event of an emergency, or if you require a second opinion or assistance intraoperatively. Clear communication with other medical and non-medical staff is important in critical situations. Tools have been developed to aid communication, such as SBAR (see Chapter 13), which is a structured method for communicating important information in critical situations.

Recently there have been many initiatives aimed at improving the human factors element of hospital care. For example, the NHS 'patient safety-first' initiative aims to change hospital culture through human factors training. This aims to create an open, just, reporting, learning, informed culture with appropriate training (Figure 6.1).

### Further reading

www.who.int/patientsafety/safesurgery/ss_checklist/en/ (accessed 22 May 2016).

# 7 Focused history

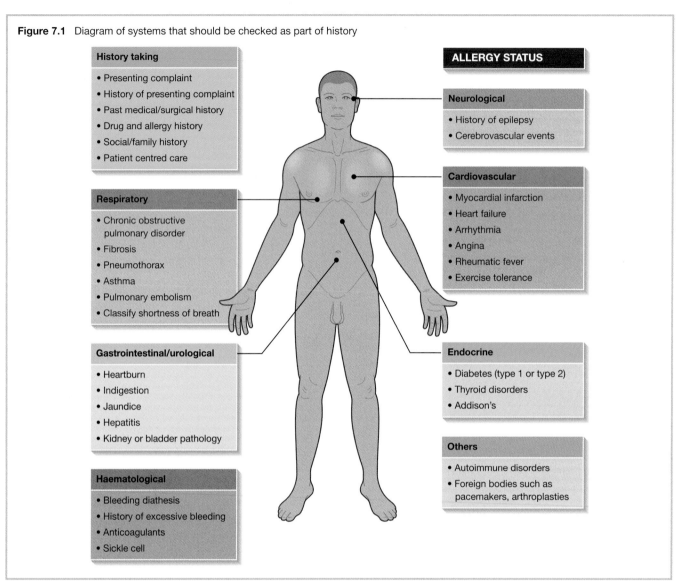

**Figure 7.1** Diagram of systems that should be checked as part of history

**History taking**

- Presenting complaint
- History of presenting complaint
- Past medical/surgical history
- Drug and allergy history
- Social/family history
- Patient centred care

**Respiratory**

- Chronic obstructive pulmonary disorder
- Fibrosis
- Pneumothorax
- Asthma
- Pulmonary embolism
- Classify shortness of breath

**Gastrointestinal/urological**

- Heartburn
- Indigestion
- Jaundice
- Hepatitis
- Kidney or bladder pathology

**Haematological**

- Bleeding diathesis
- History of excessive bleeding
- Anticoagulants
- Sickle cell

**ALLERGY STATUS**

**Neurological**

- History of epilepsy
- Cerebrovascular events

**Cardiovascular**

- Myocardial infarction
- Heart failure
- Arrhythmia
- Angina
- Rheumatic fever
- Exercise tolerance

**Endocrine**

- Diabetes (type 1 or type 2)
- Thyroid disorders
- Addison's

**Others**

- Autoimmune disorders
- Foreign bodies such as pacemakers, arthroplasties

*Minor Surgery at a Glance*, First Edition. Edited by Helen Mohan and Desmond Winter. © 2017 John Wiley & Sons, Ltd. Published 2017 by John Wiley & Sons, Ltd.

# Focused history for minor surgery

Minor surgery tends to be performed as a short stay or day case. The history and examination is an integral part of the process and will guide the procedure that is proposed and anaesthetic technique. Key considerations are whether there are any relevant features in the patient's past medical, drug, social and family history (Figure 7.1). The history is important in identifying if patients are inappropriate for day case surgery due to co-morbidity or social reasons. The presenting complaint and history of presenting complaint will vary widely dependent on the disease process and are not covered in this chapter.

## Past medical history

**Cardiovascular:** Ask the patient about previous myocardial infarction, heart failure, arrhythmias and any symptoms suggestive of angina and clarify if this occurs on exercise, at rest or at night. Ask specifically if they have a metallic valve as they may require antibiotic prophylaxis for certain procedures, or may be on anticoagulants.

**Respiratory:** Ask about any history of chronic obstructive pulmonary disease (COPD), fibrosis, pneumothorax, asthma and pulmonary embolus. Grade any shortness of breath into breathlessness at rest, on laying flat, on exertion, on climbing stairs and distance to onset of symptoms.

**Gastrointestinal:** Does the patient suffer from heartburn or severe indigestion, as this may be relevant for induction of anaesthesia if for general anaesthetic? Is there a history of liver impairment?

**Neurological:** Particularly any history of convulsions or fits.

**Endocrine:** Diabetes is common and must be asked about during a history. Clarify if the patient's diabetes is diet/tablet controlled or requiring insulin. It is helpful to know how well their diabetes is controlled or if are they prone to hypoglycaemic attacks. If the procedure requires fasting, patients with diabetes should be operated on first on the list if possible, to minimise the fasting period. Patients with diabetes also have higher risks of post-operative infection. Other endocrine conditions include Addison's and thyroid disorders.

**Haematological:** Ask about a history of excessive bleeding or bruising (e.g. following shaving or dental extraction). Ask specifically about drugs such as antiplatelets and anticoagulants, and about genetic bleeding disorders (e.g. haemophilia/von Willebrand disease and rare types). Is there any history of sickle cell disease or trait?

**Autoimmune disease:** Ask if patients are on immunosuppressants or steroids.

**Metalwork:** Does the patient have a pacemaker or any other foreign bodies such as artificial joint replacements, which could have a bearing on placement of diathermy return electrodes?

## Past surgical/anaesthetic history

Ask about any previous surgical history and what type of anaesthetic was used, for example general, spinal or local. Did they have previous hypertrophic or keloid scars? Were there any adverse reactions to anaesthetics or any post-operative nausea and vomiting (PONV)/malignant hyperthermia?

## Drug history

**Regular medication:** Particularly anti-platelet/ anti-coagulant therapy, steroids, over the counter medication. Note the correct dosage, frequency and mode of administration.

**Any known drug allergies:** Clarify the nature of the allergy or sensitivity and document. A patient's interpretation of an allergy can have a broad definition from nausea to life-threatening anaphylaxis. Ask about commonly used medical equipment and drugs such as plasters, skin preparation agents, local anaesthetic, general anaesthetic agents and antibiotics.

## Social history

• Occupation: As you can advise on disability following the procedure and time off work.
• Smoking: This will impact on wound healing and fitness for anaesthesia.
• Alcohol and recreational drug use: Clarify amount of beer/wine/spirits. How many units per day? If using recreational drugs, what type and mode of administration?
• Is there a responsible adult at home to look after them if having a day case procedure? Do they have stairs or other factors at home that may cause difficulties following the procedure?

## Family history

Ask about family history of bleeding or clotting disorders, or of reactions to anaesthetic.

## Systems review and summary

**Others:** Jaundice, hepatitis, rheumatic fever, deep vein thrombosis/pulmonary embolism.

## Patient-centred care

• Patient's perspective: How does the disease impact on them? What research have they done and what treatment would they like (if any)?
• Any particular concerns such as needle phobia?
• Discuss anaesthetic options, for example, local/regional and general anaesthesia.

## Day surgery

• The advantages of day case surgery if the patient and the procedure are suitable are that it is economical and reduces patients' exposure to hospital wards, which can induce anxiety or potentially expose them to hospital-acquired infections.
• To improve a patient's experience with day surgery requires excellent communication from hospital staff about the system and modifying the patient's previous concepts of health care.

# 8 Specimen processing and reporting

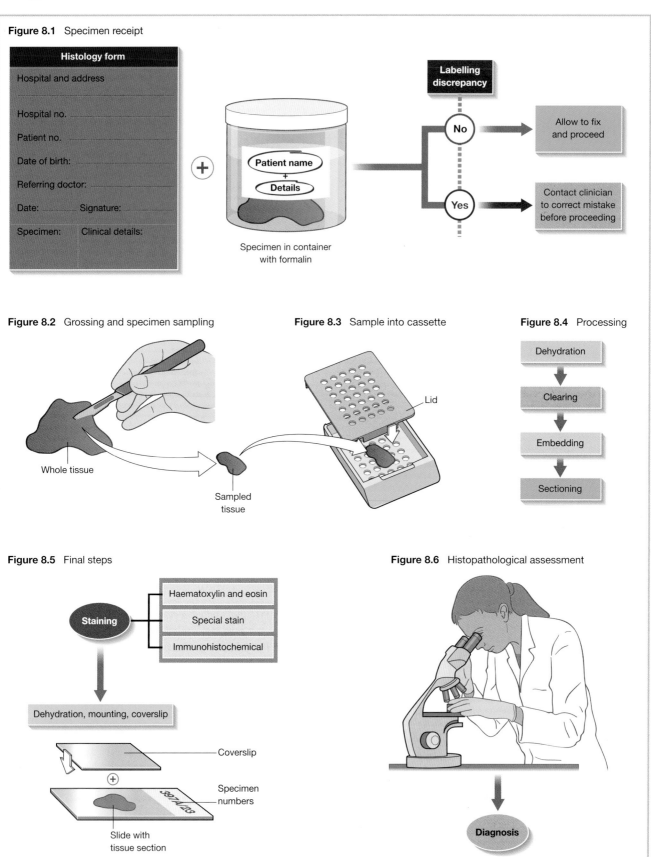

**Figure 8.1** Specimen receipt

| Histology form |
| --- |
| Hospital and address |
| Hospital no. |
| Patient no. |
| Date of birth: |
| Referring doctor: |
| Date:          Signature: |
| Specimen:     Clinical details: |

Specimen in container with formalin

Patient name
+
Details

Labelling discrepancy

No → Allow to fix and proceed

Yes → Contact clinician to correct mistake before proceeding

**Figure 8.2** Grossing and specimen sampling

Whole tissue

Sampled tissue

**Figure 8.3** Sample into cassette

Lid

**Figure 8.4** Processing

Dehydration → Clearing → Embedding → Sectioning

**Figure 8.5** Final steps

Staining
- Haematoxylin and eosin
- Special stain
- Immunohistochemical

Dehydration, mounting, coverslip

Coverslip

Specimen numbers

Slide with tissue section

**Figure 8.6** Histopathological assessment

Diagnosis

*Minor Surgery at a Glance*, First Edition. Edited by Helen Mohan and Desmond Winter. © 2017 John Wiley & Sons, Ltd. Published 2017 by John Wiley & Sons, Ltd.

## Specimen handling and labelling

When a specimen is surgically removed it is important that it is handled gently to avoid trauma caused by tearing, cautery or crushing. This damage may preclude an accurate diagnosis. Similarly, it must be placed in the appropriate solution and correctly labelled (Figure 8.1). The specimen must be placed in a secure container of appropriate size. It should be labelled with the specimen type and three patient identifiers (i.e. name, date of birth and hospital number). A histology form must accompany the specimen and contain sufficient information to enable adequate interpretation of results by the histopathologist.

### Clinical details:

• The patient's symptoms and physician's clinical impression.

### Specimen details:

• The type of specimen, site and laterality of excision.
• How the specimen was harvested (e.g. hot or cold biopsy).
• Orientation: In some cases a suture can be used to orientate the specimen (e.g. a suture at the distal end). If the specimen is pinned out on a cork board, a hand-drawn illustration describing the orientation is very useful.

When a labelling discrepancy occurs, the submitting clinician will usually be contacted to correct the error. Any specimen submission error will delay sample processing and reporting of results.

## Tissue preservation

The majority of specimens are sent to the laboratory in a fixative, which stabilises cellular composition and prevents digestion by enzymes or bacteria. Examples include formaldehyde, glutaraldehyde and alcohol. Formaldehyde is the most popular agent used for histopathology and when dissolved in water is referred to as 'formalin'. A 10% formalin solution is the optimal concentration for fixation, penetrating tissue at about one millimetre an hour. In general, biopsies are submitted for processing to permanent sections the same day as received, if they are received in formalin. Larger specimens (e.g. a mastectomy) are not processed the same day as received as they require a longer fixation period.

In some cases specimens are sent fresh (i.e. not in formalin), e.g. lymph nodes suspected to have lymphoma are examined while fresh and divided into smaller pieces for histology, flow cytometry, immunoglobulin gene rearrangement studies etc. Similarly, muscle biopsies are often sent fresh. Fresh tissue should not be allowed to dry out. Therefore, prior to fixation fresh tissue should be placed on gauze moistened with saline only. Specimens may sometimes be sent to another institution for analysis and require placement in different solutions. It is therefore wise to always check what local practice is as it may vary.

## Processing and staining of tissue

'Grossing' of histopathology specimens involves careful examination by the pathologist once the specimen is received (Figure 8.2). Following fixation, the relevant areas are sampled, placed into a cassette (Figure 8.3) and undergo a series of steps (Figure 8.4):

• Dehydration: To remove fixative and cell water.
• Clearing: To replace dehydrating fluid with clearing fluid.
• Embedding: To impregnate the tissue with liquid paraffin.
• Sectioning: To make tissue sections available for histological analysis (using an instrument with fine blades called a microtome).
• Staining: To make various components of the tissue visible by using mixtures of dyes. This includes routine staining (using the combination of haematoxylin and eosin, or the 'H&E'; stain), special stains (to stain particular structures e.g. elastin stain for vessels) or immunohistochemical stains (to detect antigens in cells e.g. oestrogen receptor expression).
• Final steps: The stained specimen is once again dehydrated, rinsed and a coverslip applied (mounted) on top of the sample to protect it (Figure 8.5). The slide can now be viewed on the microscope (Figure 8.6).

## The frozen section technique (intraoperative consultation)

Frozen section is an alternative tissue preparation technique. It is a fast histological examination done on fresh tissue, frozen in liquid nitrogen, cut in a refrigerated microtome (or cryostat) and stained with H&E. This is used, for example, where the surgeon needs to confirm a diagnosis of cancer intraoperatively or examine a tumour margin to ensure it has been adequately removed. Turnaround time should occur within 20 minutes after receipt of the tissue by the pathology laboratory.

## Stage of disease

Once cancer has been diagnosed histologically, the extent to which the cancer has spread must be assessed, a process termed 'staging'. The TNM system is one of the most widely used cancer staging systems and is based on:

• (T) Primary tumour size
• (N) Lymph node status
• (M) Metastasis.

TNM staging can be divided into a clinical ('c') and a pathologic ('p') stage, which complement each other. Clinical stage is based on the information obtained prior to surgery (i.e. physical examination, endoscopy results, etc.), while pathologic stage includes histologic information (i.e. tumour size, grade, tumour type, etc.). Other staging systems are used for various malignancies including the FIGO (International Federation of Gynaecology and Obstetrics) staging system used for gynaecological cancer or the Ann Arbor staging classification for lymphoma.

## The surgical pathology report

The pathology report is the final document that contains macroscopic details (i.e. size, weight, colour, etc.), microscopic details (i.e. tumour type, grade, margin status, etc.) and tumour stage. It may also include the results of immunohistochemical stains, special stains or molecular results (e.g. EGFR status). It is important to follow-up histology results in a timely manner to avoid delays in diagnosis and treatment.

# 9 Follow-up

**Figure 9.1** Communication with primary care

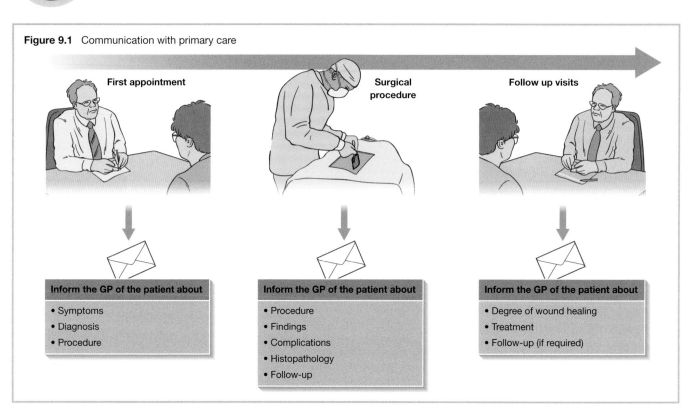

First appointment

Surgical procedure

Follow up visits

**Inform the GP of the patient about**
- Symptoms
- Diagnosis
- Procedure

**Inform the GP of the patient about**
- Procedure
- Findings
- Complications
- Histopathology
- Follow-up

**Inform the GP of the patient about**
- Degree of wound healing
- Treatment
- Follow-up (if required)

*Minor Surgery at a Glance*, First Edition. Edited by Helen Mohan and Desmond Winter. © 2017 John Wiley & Sons, Ltd. Published 2017 by John Wiley & Sons, Ltd.

# Introduction

On discharge, patients require information regarding their wound, dressings, potential complications and how to manage them. Follow-up also includes communicating with other healthcare providers, for example the patient's family doctor/general practitioner (GP). There must be a clear plan for follow-up of relevant laboratory results (Figure 9.1).

# Dressings

For information on what dressing to use, see Chapter 22. Patients need to be informed about when the dressing should be changed and when they can shower.

# Analgesia

## What kind of medicines can you prescribe to your patient?

• Step 1: Non-opioid analgesics: paracetamol and/or non-steroidal anti-inflammatory drugs (NSAIDs).
• Step 2: Weak opioids, e.g. a combination of paracetamol and codeine, or tramadol hydrochloride.
• Step 3: Strong opioid, e.g. morphine, oxycodone.

Generally, the strong opioids are not needed for minor operations – if a patient requires these strong analgesics, consider whether it is really appropriate to discharge the patient and decide on a case-by-case basis. A proton pump inhibitor may be advisable if discharging a patient on NSAIDs. Consider contraindications to the above medications prior to choosing to prescribe them. For example, NSAIDs may be contraindicated in patients with renal failure, asthma, bleeding disorders or previous peptic ulcer disease.

# Complications

For a detailed description of complications see Chapter 48.

## Information to give patients about complications

1 Bleeding: Apply pressure manually. Where possible, elevate the bleeding area. Apply a fresh dressing when the bleeding stops. If the bleeding is profuse or not settling after 10 minutes, seek urgent medical attention.

2 Infection: If the patient sees signs of infection – such as redness, heat, tenderness, discharge or loss of function – they should seek medical attention.
3 Wound dehiscence: If the patient notices the wound 'coming apart', they should seek medical attention.
4 Swelling: Post-operative swellings may be a seroma (collection of serous fluid), haematoma (collection of blood), or an abscess. If the patient develops a significant post-operative swelling, they should seek medical attention.

# Follow-up plan

## When and where?

• Removal of sutures/clips:
  • Head and face: after 4–8 days
  • Trunk and limbs: after 10–15 days.
• For uncomplicated and clean wounds, the public health nurse and/or the GP can usually provide follow-up and removal of sutures/clips. For complicated wounds (closure by secondary intention, contaminated wounds, high risk of infection or complications) an outpatient or dressing clinic follow-up may be required.

## Discussion of the results

• Depending on local policies and arrangements, follow-up may be in the outpatients, in a virtual outpatients or with the GP/primary healthcare provider.
• Follow-up of histopathology results must be arranged in a timely fashion. When a lesion is suspicious, ensure urgent follow-up. Consider discussing with the pathologist if you have a high suspicion of malignancy and keep the patient's details to check histology reports.

# Information for GP letter

1 Name, date of birth and hospital number of the patient
2 Short summary and indication for surgery
3 Surgical site
4 Date of the surgery
5 Type of surgery and if relevant, complications
6 Histopathology results if available (if not available mention that they are pending and who will follow them up)
7 Date of removal of sutures or clips, if needed
8 Date of the appointments arranged (dressing clinic, outpatients, etc.)
9 Mention if a follow-up by the GP is requested or not.

# 10 Anaphylaxis

**Figure 10.1** Anaphylaxis algorithm

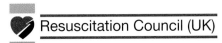 Resuscitation Council (UK)

## Anaphylaxis algorithm

**Anaphylactic reaction?**

**Airway, Breathing, Circulation, Disability, Exposure**

**Diagnosis** - look for:
- Acute onset of illness
- Life-threatening Airway and/or Breathing and/or Circulation problems[1]
- And usually skin changes

- **Call for help**
- Lie patient flat
- Raise patient's legs

**Adrenaline[2]**

**When skills and equipment available:**
- Establish airway
- High flow oxygen
- IV fluid challenge[3]
- Chlorphenamine[4]
- Hydrocortisone[5]

**Monitor:**
- Pulse oximetry
- ECG
- Blood pressure

**[1] Life-threatening problems:**

| | |
|---|---|
| **Airway:** | swelling, hoarseness, stridor |
| **Breathing:** | rapid breathing, wheeze, fatigue, cyanosis, $SpO_2$ < 92%, confusion |
| **Circulation:** | pale, clammy, low blood pressure, faintness, drowsy/coma |

**[2] Adrenaline** *(give IM unless experienced with IV adrenaline)*
IM doses of 1:1000 adrenaline (repeat after 5 min if no better)

- Adult      500 micrograms IM (0.5 mL)
- Child more than 12 years: 500 micrograms IM (0.5 mL)
- Child 6 -12 years:      300 micrograms IM (0.3 mL)
- Child less than 6 years:      150 micrograms IM (0.15 mL)

Adrenaline IV to be given **only by experienced specialists**
Titrate: Adults 50 micrograms; Children 1 microgram/kg

**[3] IV fluid challenge:**

Adult - 500 – 1000 mL
Child - crystalloid 20 mL/kg

Stop IV colloid
if this might be the cause
of anaphylaxis

| | **[4] Chlorphenamine** (IM or slow IV) | **[5] Hydrocortisone** (IM or slow IV) |
|---|---|---|
| Adult or child more than 12 years | 10 mg | 200 mg |
| Child 6 - 12 years | 5 mg | 100 mg |
| Child 6 months to 6 years | 2.5 mg | 50 mg |
| Child less than 6 months | 250 micrograms/kg | 25 mg |

March 2008

*Minor Surgery at a Glance*, First Edition. Edited by Helen Mohan and Desmond Winter. © 2017 John Wiley & Sons, Ltd. Published 2017 by John Wiley & Sons, Ltd.

# Anaphylaxis

Anaphylaxis is a severe, life-threatening, generalised hypersensitivity reaction. The term anaphylaxis encompasses both 'anaphylactic shock' and 'severe allergic reaction'.

Anaphylaxis is caused by IgE-mediated mast cell degranulation with systemic release of histamine. Histamine causes vasodilatation, bronchoconstriction and extravasation of intravascular fluid.

Common causes of drug-induced anaphylaxis in the perioperative environment are paralytic agents such as suxamethonium, atracurium and rocuronium. Other notable agents are antibiotics, latex and colloid fluids.

## Recognition of anaphylaxis

Suspect anaphylaxis in a patient who develops any of:
- Sudden deterioration in clinical condition
- Sudden airway, breathing or circulatory compromise
- Sudden skin or mucosal changes.

Anaphylaxis occurs quickly – most cardiac arrests from anaphylaxis to injected substances occur within 20 minutes of initial exposure.

### Life-threatening features (indications for adrenaline)

**Airway:** Tongue or lip swelling, stridor, hoarseness.

**Breathing:** Cyanosis, confusion, respiratory distress.

**Circulation:** Collapse, shock, bradycardia.

⚑ Call for critical care support immediately if you suspect anaphylaxis, as intubation may be necessary.

## Medical interventions for anaphylaxis

### Adrenaline (epinephrine)

Adrenaline acts within seconds of administration and should be prioritised over all other treatments when anaphylaxis occurs.

Adrenaline causes vasoconstriction and reduced extravasation ($\alpha_1$), increased myocardial contractility ($\beta_1$), bronchodilation and mast cell inhibition ($\beta_2$).

Adrenaline in anaphylaxis should be given intramuscularly (IM).

Pre-filled adrenaline syringes found on cardiac arrest carts contain 1000 micrograms of adrenaline in 10 mL (1 in 10 000 solution). This is not suitable for intramuscular injection.

Intravenous adrenaline is not recommended for anaphylaxis outside critical care areas and for those not experienced in its use.

### Antihistamines

Antihistamines block $H_1$ histamine receptors, and act within minutes of parenteral administration. All currently available parenteral $H_1$ blockers are first-generation, 'sedating' antihistamines. Chlorphenamine (chlorpheniramine) is typically used for anaphylaxis.

### Steroids

Steroids may reduce the duration of a prolonged reaction, or prevent one recurring. The onset of action of intravenous steroids is far slower than other treatments for anaphylaxis. Steroids should not be prioritised over other treatments. Hydrocortisone is typically used.

## Surgical interventions for anaphylaxis

Laryngeal oedema leading to airway obstruction and cardiac arrest is a major complication of anaphylaxis. In these circumstances, swelling may prevent orotracheal intubation and a life-saving surgical airway is needed. A simple method to perform a surgical airway is described here.
- Locate cricothyroid membrane with non-dominant hand.
- Vertically incise skin from thyroid cartilage prominence inferiorly for 6 cm.
- Puncture the cricothyroid membrane with the scalpel.
- Transfer scalpel to non-dominant hand, slide a bougie or intubating catheter pointed inferiorly into the trachea.
- Remove the scalpel.
- Slide a size 5 or 6 cuffed endotracheal tube along the bougie through the incision site into the trachea.
- Remove the bougie.
- Inflate balloon to at least 5 cm air and ventilate through the endotracheal tube with a bag-valve mask.

## Follow-up for anaphylaxis

### In hospital

Patients who develop anaphylaxis should be observed for at least 6 hours and reviewed by a senior clinician prior to discharge.

### After discharge

All patients with anaphylaxis should be referred for follow-up with an immunologist. Not all patients who had anaphylaxis need to carry an adrenaline auto-injector for self-administration ('pen'). Typical recommendations for prescription of an adrenaline auto-injector include:
- Anaphylaxis to food (especially nuts), insect or arachnid venom-these are substances that are difficult to avoid
- Anaphylaxis that required intensive care-level support.

### Mast cell tryptase

Mast cell tryptase is used to confirm the diagnosis of an anaphylactic reaction in equivocal cases. It is *not* performed routinely on patients with anaphylaxis, particularly when the diagnosis is not in doubt.

Samples for mast cell tryptase should be taken at the following intervals: as soon as safely possible after onset of symptoms; 1–2 hours after onset of symptoms; and more than 24 hours after symptoms have resolved.

### *Further reading*

Nel L, Eren E. Peri-operative anaphylaxis. *British Journal of Clinical Pharmacology* 2011; 71(5): 647–658.

UK resuscitation council. Anaphylaxis – Guideline for Healthcare Providers, 2008. https://www.resus.org.uk/anaphylaxis/emergency-treatment-of-anaphylactic-reactions/

# 11 Emergencies and resuscitation

It is important that staff in units undertaking any form of surgical procedure are appropriately trained in resuscitation. For a patient without signs of life, the Advanced Life Support (ALS) cardiac arrest algorithm is followed as shown in Figure 11.1. For a patient with signs of life, a structured approach based on ALS principles is performed. For further information on cardiac arrest and resuscitation, please consult your local training centre, the American Heart Association website or Resuscitation Council website, and the ALS/Advanced Cardiac Life Support (ACLS) provider manuals.

## Advanced life support algorithm

**Figure 11.1** In-hospital resuscitation

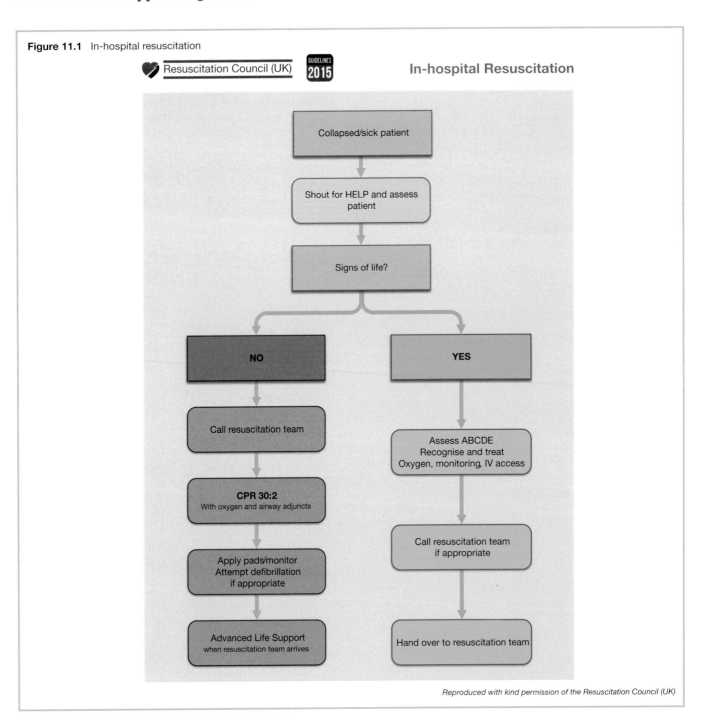

Resuscitation Council (UK)  GUIDELINES 2015  **In-hospital Resuscitation**

Collapsed/sick patient

Shout for HELP and assess patient

Signs of life?

NO

YES

Call resuscitation team

CPR 30:2
With oxygen and airway adjuncts

Apply pads/monitor
Attempt defibrillation
if appropriate

Advanced Life Support
when resuscitation team arrives

Assess ABCDE
Recognise and treat
Oxygen, monitoring, IV access

Call resuscitation team
if appropriate

Hand over to resuscitation team

*Reproduced with kind permission of the Resuscitation Council (UK)*

# 12 Audit and practice

**Figure 12.1** Principles of clinical governance

Practice standards: Continuing professional development, code of practice

Accountability

Clinical effectiveness: research and review

Open culture

**Clinical governance**

Audit

Systems to monitor risk, reduce risk and learn from mistakes

Managing risk by developing guidelines, protocols, implementation strategies

Education and training

**Figure 12.2** The audit cycle

1. Identify problem

5. Implement change

2. Set standards

4. Compare to standards

3. Collect data on current practice

## Clinical governance

Clinical governance (Figure 12.1) is important in modern surgical practice. Clinical governance is the framework through which healthcare providers are accountable for the quality, safety and experience of patients in the care they have delivered. It involves identifying clinical standards of care and measuring them to demonstrate that these standards are being achieved. It includes activities like audit, education and training, clinical effectiveness, research and development, openness and risk management.

## Audit

### Key point
Audit is a process of continuous quality improvement, and a key component of clinical governance.

Performing clinical audit is a requirement for medical registration in many jurisdictions, as part of continuing professional development. Surgical audit is important in identifying areas for improvement in practice and proving continuous quality improvement. The process involves evaluating outcomes against specific criteria, implementing change to improve outcomes, and re-auditing.

Aspects of practice that may be audited include:
- Outcomes following specific procedures
- The process of care
- Waiting times, follow-up
- Patient satisfaction.

The audit cycle (Figure 12.2) consists of the following:

**1 Identifying the problem** or condition to be audited.
For example, an audit of incomplete excision rates following excision of basal cell carcinoma (BCC).

**2 Set standards**
For example, British Association of Dermatology Guidelines – incomplete excision occurs in 4.7–6.0% of BCCs in plastic surgery units in the UK.

**3 Collect data**
For example, review pathology records and operation notes from all BCC excised in the past year in the unit and then calculate the rate of incomplete excision.

**4 Compare to standards**
For example, if you found your unit had a 10% rate of incomplete excision, compare this to the 4.7–6% rate in the standard you are auditing against. Look carefully to see if there are any systematic differences in the patient cohort and management that may act as confounding factors that may need to be controlled for in the analysis.

**5 Implement change**
For example, print a copy of the guidelines and laminate them and leave them in theatre or the minor operations room, implement an education and awareness programme among the surgical team to make them aware of the shortcomings of the unit and educate them on what current guidelines are.

The next step is in many ways the most important and the most difficult – go back after a period of time and re-audit to 'close the audit loop' to see if the changes have been effective in modifying clinical practice to meet the set standards. If not, implement change again and re-audit.

### Further reading
http://www.hqip.org.uk/resources/hqip-clinical-audit-programme-guidance/

http://www.hse.ie/eng/about/Who/qualityandpatientsafety/Clinical_Governance/CG_docs/clingovinformleafletFeb2012.pdf

*Minor Surgery at a Glance*, First Edition. Edited by Helen Mohan and Desmond Winter. © 2017 John Wiley & Sons, Ltd. Published 2017 by John Wiley & Sons, Ltd.

# 13 Communication and conflict resolution

**Figure 13.1** Effective communication expands across primary, secondary and social care to ensure the patient is at the centre of care

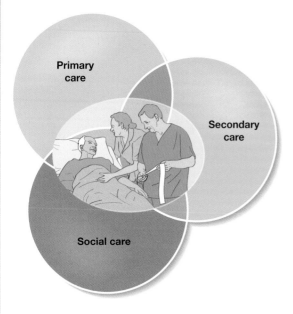

Primary care

Secondary care

Social care

**Figure 13.2** Situation–Background–Assessment–Recommendation (SBAR system)

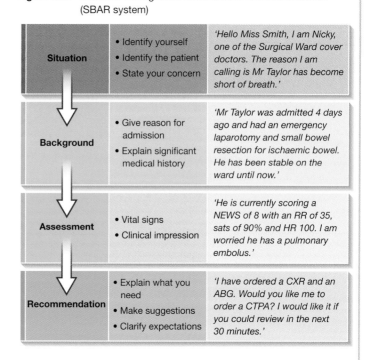

| | | |
|---|---|---|
| **Situation** | • Identify yourself<br>• Identify the patient<br>• State your concern | *'Hello Miss Smith, I am Nicky, one of the Surgical Ward cover doctors. The reason I am calling is Mr Taylor has become short of breath.'* |
| **Background** | • Give reason for admission<br>• Explain significant medical history | *'Mr Taylor was admitted 4 days ago and had an emergency laparotomy and small bowel resection for ischaemic bowel. He has been stable on the ward until now.'* |
| **Assessment** | • Vital signs<br>• Clinical impression | *'He is currently scoring a NEWS of 8 with an RR of 35, sats of 90% and HR 100. I am worried he has a pulmonary embolus.'* |
| **Recommendation** | • Explain what you need<br>• Make suggestions<br>• Clarify expectations | *'I have ordered a CXR and an ABG. Would you like me to order a CTPA? I would like it if you could review in the next 30 minutes.'* |

**Figure 13.3** Factors that lead to conflict in the healthcare system

**Needs**
'I also have reponsibilities to my family that I need to meet'

**Structures**
'This public healthcare system does not work for physicians'

**Relationships**
'I don't feel the consultant actually respects me'

**Factors leading to conflicts**

**Emotions**
'I feel undervalued in my organisation'

**Communication**
'How can the managers just send an email about that? Why did they not talk to me directly?'

**History**
'I have voiced my concerns about these issues before and still nothing has changed'

**Figure 13.4** Strategies to deal with aggression

Refrain from raising your voice and remain calm

Put some distance between yourself and the aggressor

Remain neutral and non-judgemental

**Dealing with aggression**

Protect yourself: bring a chaperone

Allow them time to have their say, but if getting no resolve apologise that you will have to leave the situation

Debrief after the incident with your senior (particularly if you are upset)

**Table 13.1** Types of conflict with examples and suggested strategies to deal with them

| Conflict type | Example | Strategy to deal with this |
|---|---|---|
| **Interpersonal** | Mr X believes we need to operate on the patient, but Mr T is refusing to anaesthetise him. The two consultants are now shouting at each other. | • Listen to others and recognise different opinions will exist<br>• Learn to compromise with others<br>• In this scenario someone may need to mediate to allow each consultant to have their view heard |
| **Intrapersonal** | You have started a surgical training job but feel you are not coping and would prefer to become a General Practitioner, but you're worried you'll let people down. | • Ask others what they would do<br>• If you're not coping speak to your supervisor who may be able to offer you a solution<br>• Don't let the decision become overwhelming leading to depression or anxiety that will affect you doing your job at present |
| **Intragroup** | Dr S is a keen surgeon and will leave his colleague Dr D on the ward to do the discharge summaries and cannulas while he goes off to theatre. Dr D appreciates Dr S needs to fill out his logbook but feels disgruntled she is always left to do the mundane tasks. | • Embrace the fact that your team has different personalities in it<br>• Ensure every team member feels valued and can contribute their strengths to the group<br>• Ensure everyone is doing their share of the mundane tasks |
| **Intergroup** | Surgical specialty X thinks that surgical speciality Y gets more theatre time than they do. They believe management are favouring surgical speciality Y and as a consequence are starting to resent speciality Y and morale is becoming low. | • Ensure constant communication between teams<br>• Have regular meetings to look at figures relating to theatre usage, inviting everyone who is affected by its use<br>• Give people time to talk about their frustrations and offer solutions |

*Minor Surgery at a Glance*, First Edition. Edited by Helen Mohan and Desmond Winter. © 2017 John Wiley & Sons, Ltd. Published 2017 by John Wiley & Sons, Ltd.

# Communication skills

Communication skills form the basis of good patient care. Communication between doctors and patients has evolved over the years from a paternal to a partnership model with regulatory bodies now actively encouraging doctors to work in partnership with patients. Communication with patients often extends to their family, with the patient's consent. Our multi-disciplinary healthcare system requires doctors to communicate effectively with colleagues from other medical specialties, nursing staff and allied health professionals. The inter-link between primary, secondary and social care needs to be robust to ensure patient centred care. It is communication that underpins this system (Figure 13.1). Lack of effective communication creates situations where medical errors can occur. Medical indemnity organisations consistently cite communication issues as the commonest cause for medical litigation. With changing shift patterns, handover of patients can occur up to four times a day. A structured, thorough handover with excellent communication between teams is pertinent to ensure patient safety.

## What are the different types of communication?

**1 Verbal:** Verbal communication is the main method used in the healthcare setting. Doctors will communicate with patients & relatives, with each other on ward rounds or when taking referrals which can either be in person or over the telephone. Verbal communication is also the main method of communication in the operating theatre.

**2 Non-verbal:** Body language plays an enormous role in effective communication. Up to 93% of communication is affected by body language, tone and attitude, with only 7% being related to the actual words said.

**3 Visual:** Drawing diagrams or showing the patient their investigations (e.g. scan pictures) can help reinforce key messages.

**4 Written:** Written communication is used when patients are seen in the outpatient clinic or are being discharged from hospital. It is often the only way the General Practitioner will become aware that their patient has been seen in secondary care and the plan for further management. Leaflets on procedures and conditions can be given to patients to re-enforce what has been explained during the consultation.

## Structured methods of communication

### Situation–Background–Assessment–Recommendation (SBAR)

Due to the differences in nursing and medical training, often nurses and doctors have different communication styles; nursing staff tend to be more descriptive, whereas doctors are taught to be more concise. The SBAR system (Figure 13.2) provides a framework to communicate information concisely about a patient's condition, to highlight an issue requiring the clinician's immediate attention and action.

## Key tips for effective communication

✓ **Get the setting right**: If you are breaking bad news ensure you have a quiet room where you will not be interrupted.

✓ **Listen**: When taking a history from the patient allow them to speak without any interruptions for the first minute – you will gain a lot of information from this.

✓ **Be interested and focus your attention on them**: Do not be distracted by what is going on around you. Actively show that you are listening to their concerns.

✓ **Clarity of speech**: Be clear and concise in your information. Use phrases and detail that is easily understandable.

✓ **Give the patient time to ask questions** and check for their understanding at regular intervals.

# Conflict resolution

Conflict occurs in the healthcare setting frequently and is caused by our needs being unmet or because our needs are inconsistent or in opposition to the needs of others (Figure 13.3). Due to the complexity of our healthcare system often conflict can occur at multiple levels at the same time. Conflict can occur between colleagues or between patient and doctor.

## Types of conflict

There are four main types of conflict (Table 13.1).

**1 Interpersonal** – conflict between two individuals.
**2 Intrapersonal** – occurs within an individual.
**3 Intragroup** – conflict among individuals within a team.
**4 Intergroup** – occurs when a misunderstanding arises between teams within an organisation.

## Consequences of conflict in the healthcare system

Conflict can result in adverse effects on individuals and on the healthcare system. This can result in *lost productivity* – if the employee is spending their time attempting to resolve conflict then their energy is not being placed into getting their jobs done; *lost employees and low morale* – if tensions run high for too long people may start to become absent from work or leave all their jobs altogether; burnout – conflict can also create a negative work ecosystem that can lead to burnout; *litigation and complaints* – from patient or relatives who do not feel they received resolution to their conflicts.

## Key techniques in conflict resolution

The goal of conflict resolution is de-escalation. It is important to speak in a clear way with a measured and level tone. Do not lose your temper but do not afraid to be firm when required.

**1 Ensure your own safety** – make sure that you have a clear path to the door in order to make quick exit if required. Consider having another member of your team with you.

**2 Listen before you talk** – allow the other person to voice their point of view.

**3 Acknowledge that there is an issue** – this reinforces that you are listening.

**4 Explore potential solutions** – find out what the other party wants done.

**5 Agree a mutually acceptable solution** – compromise is often the key to taking conflict forward.

If these techniques fail and the interaction begins to escalate towards verbal or physical aggression, you must remove yourself to a safe distance at the earliest opportunity (Figure 13.4).

### Further reading

http://www.institute.nhs.uk/quality_and_service_improvement_tools/quality_and_service_improvement_tools/sbar_-_situation_-_background_-_assessment_-_recommendation.html (accessed 20 June 2016)

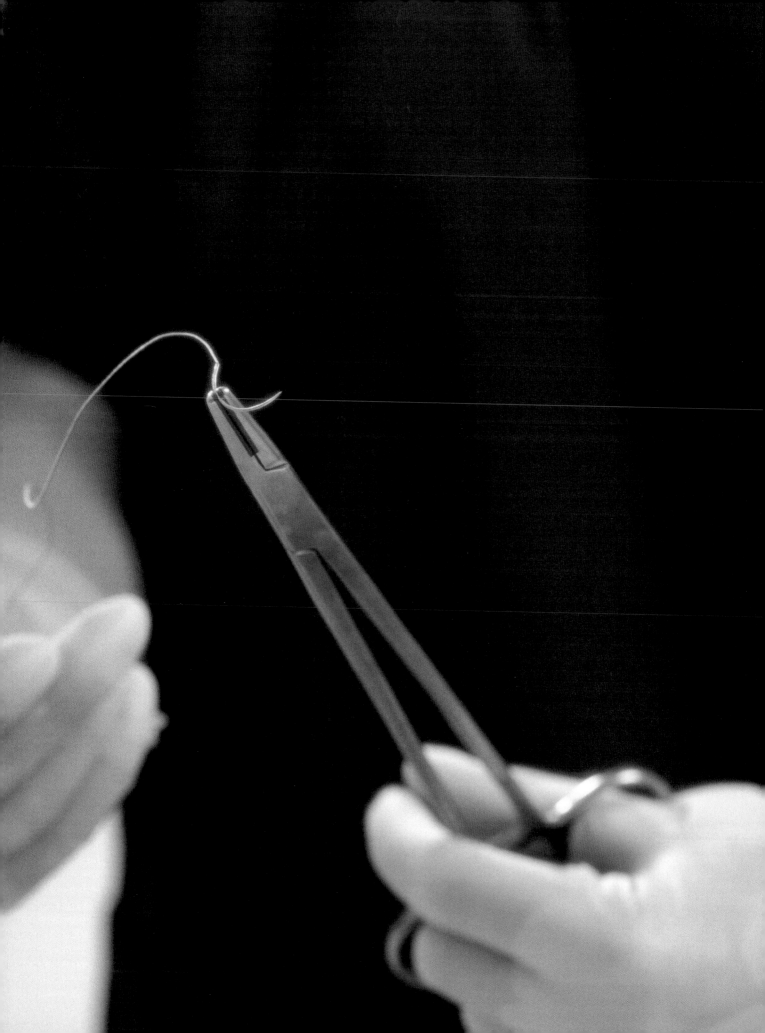

# Basic pain control and anaesthesia

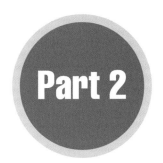

**Part 2**

## Chapters

# 14 Local anaesthesia

**Table 14.1** Duration of action of local anaesthetic agents

| Drug | Onset | Duration of action |
|---|---|---|
| Lignocaine | Rapid | 1–2 hours |
| Bupivacaine | Slow | 6–16 hours (PNBs) |
| Levobupivacaine | Slow | 6–16 hours (PNBs) |
| Cocaine | 1–5 mins | <30 mins |
| Amethocaine | 3 mins | 30–60 mins |
| Ropivacaine | Moderate | 8–13 hours (PNBs) |

PNBs denotes when used for peripheral nerve blocks

**Table 14.2** Doses of local anaesthetic drugs

| Drug | Mg/kg without adrenaline | Mg/kg with adrenaline |
|---|---|---|
| Amethocaine | 1 | 1.5 |
| Lignocaine | 4 | 7 |
| Ropivacaine | 2 | 3 |
| Bupivacaine | 2 | 3 |
| Levobupivacaine | 2 | 3 |

**Box 14.1** Treatment for local anaesthetic toxicity

**If the patient suffers local anaesthetic toxicity what should I do?**

- Stop injecting
- Call for help and administer oxygen
- Obtain IV access if not already present
- Management of local anaesthetic toxicity is largely supportive – maintaining airway, breathing and circulation
- The only specific therapy is the use of *Lipidrescue*. (full details are available on the AAGBI website)

## What is a local anaesthetic?

Local anaesthetic (LA) agents are drugs that cause reversible loss of pain perception by blocking Na+ (sodium) channels in nerve tissue. They can be administered by a number of routes, including:

- Topical: for example, amethocaine or eutectic mixture of local anaesthetic (EMLA)
- Infiltration, for example, lignocaine, bupivacaine
- Field block: for example, transversus abdominis block (TAP)
- Regional anaesthesia (nerve block): for example, brachial plexus block
- Neuraxial anaesthesia: for example, subarachnoid or epidural anaesthesia.

In general, field blocks, regional and neuraxial anaesthesia are administered by anaesthetists; however, LA infiltration and the use of LAs for ring blocks and other simple techniques are practiced more widely.

*Minor Surgery at a Glance*, First Edition. Edited by Helen Mohan and Desmond Winter. © 2017 John Wiley & Sons, Ltd. Published 2017 by John Wiley & Sons, Ltd.

EMLA is a 50:50 mixture of lignocaine and prilocaine. It is used topically for dermal anaesthesia – it accumulates in the dermis and epidermis. This can be useful prior to cannulation and also prior to infiltration of LA solutions.

**Pharmacology:** LAs are divided into two categories – esters or amides, depending on their structure. Cocaine, procaine and amethocaine are esters. Bupivacaine, lignocaine, ropivacaine, levobupivacaine and prilocaine are amide LAs. Most LAs are weak bases that are lipid soluble, diffuse into neurons and become ionised and thus bind reversibly to the sodium channels, preventing nerve conduction and thereby preventing nociception. Half-lives and times to onset of action vary, for example, lignocaine has a rapid onset of action and a half-life of 1–2 hours, while bupivacaine can take 30–40 minutes for maximum effect and has a half-life of up to 4 hours (Table 14.1). Bupivacaine and levobupivacaine are isomers of each other (mirror images at a molecular level) – much like right- and left-handed gloves. This results in slightly different properties. Levobupivacaine is less cardiotoxic than bupivacaine if given IV inadvertently, or at high doses. See Table 14.2 for doses.

## Safety considerations
### What are the side effects?

1 Local anaesthetic toxicity can occur due to either excessive dosage, or accidental intravenous administration. LA toxicity mainly affects the central nervous system (CNS) and cardiovascular system (CVS). Inadvertent intravenous (IV) administration of LA instead of subcutaneously (SC) can result in cardiac arrest. Early warning signs of toxicity are numbness around the mouth and a buzzing sensation in the ears. Generally, neurotoxicity precedes cardiovascular collapse. Confusion and agitation can proceed to seizures, coma and respiratory arrest. Continued administration at this point may proceed to hypotension, bradycardia and cardiac arrest. See Box 14.1 for treatment.
2 Direct or indirect nerve damage – compression or intraneural injection.
3 Reaction to additives – allergy to preservatives or cardiovascular effects of added vasoconstrictors.
4 Methaemoglobinaemia – this is an important adverse effect of prilocaine (e.g. in EMLA) that occurs most often if it is used in small infants and in large doses.

### What equipment/monitors should I have?

Oxygen, standard monitoring and resuscitation equipment should be available. Verbal communication is also important. A patient that is not responding may have lost airway reflexes or be suffering cardiovascular collapse.

### What are the contraindications to local anaesthesia?

**Absolute:** Patient allergy and patient refusal. Patient allergy (this is rather rare – most alleged 'allergies' to LA are as a result of the adrenaline administered with the LA, which can cause palpitations and light-headedness. True allergy to LA is quite unusual and is usually a reaction to the preservatives in the solution. Allergy to *p*-aminobenzoic acid (PABA) – a metabolite of ester LAs – however, has been described. Note this is also a component of sunscreen.

**Relative:** Uncooperative and confused patient or infection at the proposed administration site. LA is less likely to be effective in this instance as the acidic environment renders it less ionised. Also, increased blood flow in an infected site increases the rate at which the drug is eliminated.

**Anticoagulation:** Depending on the degree of anticoagulation, it may be unwise to administer LA or to carry out an operative procedure.

## How do I inject local anaesthetic safely?

Ensure you have completed an adequate history and examination. Ensure appropriate equipment and personnel (as above) are available. Work out your maximum doses prior to starting. Obtain consent from the patient explaining what you are doing and why. Prepare the skin with antiseptic. A small needle (25–27G) should be used to raise a skin wheal first. Administer slowly (low pressure injection) to decrease pain on injection. Pain is caused by both pH of the solution and from tissue expansion. The addition of sodium bicarbonate to lignocaine may also decrease pain on injection. However, the addition of sodium bicarbonate to bupivacaine causes the LA to precipitate. Always aspirate prior to injection to prevent IV administration. Proceed to a 23G needle for further infiltration, still administering slowly. Wait an appropriate period of time before testing the block. Always check that anaesthesia is adequate prior to proceeding.

## Adrenaline

Adrenaline can be added to LA solutions to prolong their duration of action, cause vasoconstriction at the site and thus better operating conditions/less blood loss, to intensify the effect of the block and to allow the use of higher doses (reduced blood flow gives slower absorption into the bloodstream).

Adrenaline should never be used for blocks where end arteries provide blood supply to an area, for example penile blocks and digital/ring blocks. It is important to bear in mind that the adrenaline is systemically absorbed and this may result in myocardial ischaemia in patients with ischaemic heart disease. Tachycardia associated with LAs containing adrenaline may be as a result of IV injection. If this occurs, the injection should be stopped. Adrenaline used in conjunction with cocaine (a potent vasoconstrictor) can precipitate fatal tachyarrhythmias.

### *Further reading*

Australian and New Zealand College of Anaesthetists (ANZCA). *Guidelines for Health Practitioners Administering Local Anaesthesia.* http://www.anzca.edu.au/documents/ps37-2013-guidelines-for-health-practitioners-admi (accessed 24 June 2016).

Cave G, Harrop-Griffiths W, Harvey M, et al. (AAGBI Working Group). *AAGBI Safety Guideline: Management of Severe Local Anaesthetic Toxicity.* Association of Anaesthetists of Great Britain and Ireland 2010. https://www.aagbi.org/sites/default/files/la_toxicity_2010_0.pdf (accessed 24 June 2016).

NYSORA – New York School for Regional Anaesthesia. http://www.nysora.com/regional-anesthesia/foundations-of-ra/3075-toxicity-of-local-anesthetics.html (accessed 24 June 2016).

Weinberg G. Lipid rescue resuscitation from local anaesthetic cardiac toxicity. *Toxicological Reviews* 2006; 25 (3): 139–145.

# 15 Sedation

**Table 15.1** Contraindications to sedation

| Absolute contraindication | Relative contraindication | Precautions |
|---|---|---|
| • Patient refusal<br>• History of allergic reaction to the drugs being used | • Not adequately fasted<br>• Difficult airway/intubation<br>• Significant co-morbid medical conditions – ASA class III or greater | • Extremes of age<br>• Long procedures<br>• Morbid obesity |

**Table 15.2** ASA score

| Grade I | A normal healthy patient |
|---|---|
| Grade II | A patient with mild systemic disease |
| Grade III | A patient with severe systemic disease |
| Grade IV | A patient with severe systemic disease that is a constant threat to life |
| Grade V | A moribund patient who is not expected to survive without the operation |

**Table 15.3** Airway assessment

| History | Physical examination |
|---|---|
| • Previous difficult intubation or mask ventilation<br>• Advanced rheumatoid arthritis<br>• Down syndrome – trisomy 21<br>• History of snoring, stridor or sleep apnoea<br>• History of airway surgery | • Morbid obesity<br>• Dysmorphic facial features<br>• Micrognathia or retrognathia<br>• Prominent upper incisors ("buck teeth")<br>• High arched palate<br>• Mallampati class > 2<br>• Reduced mouth opening, short neck and limited neck extension |

**Table 15.4** Mallampati score

| Mallampati classification | |
|---|---|
| Class 1 | Visualisaton of soft palate, fauces, uvula, anterior and posterior pillars |
| Class 2 | Visualisation of soft palate, fauces and uvula |
| Class 3 | Visualisation of soft palate and base of uvula |
| Class 4 | Soft palate not visible at all |

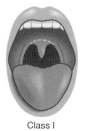 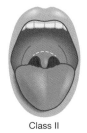 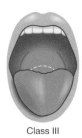 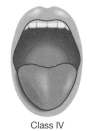

Class I     Class II     Class III     Class IV

**Table 15.5** Preoperative fasting guidelines

| Type of food ingested | Time for fasting in hours |
|---|---|
| Clear liquids | 2 |
| Breast milk | 4 |
| Infant formula | 6 |
| Non-human milk | 6 |
| Light meal | 6 |

**Table 15.6** Modified Ramsay sedation score

| 1 | Anxious |
|---|---|
| 2 | Awake and tranquil |
| 3 | Drowsy – responds easily to verbal commands |
| 4 | Asleep – brisk purposeful response to tactile stimulus |
| 5 | Asleep – minimal response to tactile or auditory stimulus |
| 6 | Asleep – no response |

*Minor Surgery at a Glance*, First Edition. Edited by Helen Mohan and Desmond Winter. © 2017 John Wiley & Sons, Ltd. Published 2017 by John Wiley & Sons, Ltd.

# Sedation and analgesia

Minor surgical procedures are routinely performed either under local anaesthesia or sedation provided by either the surgical team or an anaesthetist. The administration of sedation and/or analgesia is to ensure that the patient has a comfortable, safe and pleasant experience. However, there is a risk of serious complications with sedation. It is recognised that most adverse events that occur during sedation are preventable and hence it is imperative for the sedationist to undergo appropriate training and education to conduct safe sedation and to acquire the necessary resuscitation skills. This chapter focuses on the principles and the conduct of safe sedation and analgesia. Procedural sedation and analgesia is the term used to describe the use of sedative – hypnotic drugs and/or analgesics – to facilitate the safe conduct of a diagnostic or therapeutic procedure. This concept recognises that sedation is a continuum and patients can rapidly move between different planes of sedation and that the level of sedation required varies between individuals and the procedure performed. Typically, the drug or combinations of drugs selected allow the patient to maintain their protective airway reflexes.

# Levels of sedation and analgesia

The American Society of Anesthesiologists (ASA) has defined four levels of sedation.

### Level I: Mild sedation or anxiolysis

'A drug-induced state during which patients respond normally to verbal commands. Although cognitive function and coordination may be impaired, ventilatory and cardiovascular functions are unaffected'.

### Level II: Moderate sedation/analgesia or conscious sedation

'A drug-induced depression of consciousness during which patients respond purposefully to verbal commands, either alone or accompanied by light tactile stimulation. No interventions are required to maintain a patent airway, and spontaneous ventilation is adequate. Cardiovascular function is usually maintained'.

### Level III: Deep sedation/analgesia

'A drug-induced depression of consciousness during which patients cannot be easily aroused but respond purposefully following repeated or painful stimulation. The ability to independently maintain ventilatory function may be impaired. Patients may require assistance in maintaining a patent airway, and spontaneous ventilation may be inadequate. Cardiovascular function is usually maintained'.

### Level IV: General anaesthesia

'A drug-induced loss of consciousness during which patients are not arousable, even by painful stimulation. The ability to independently maintain ventilatory function is often impaired. Patients often require assistance in maintaining a patent airway, and positive pressure ventilation may be required because of depressed spontaneous ventilation or drug-induced depression of neuromuscular function. Cardiovascular function may be impaired'.

# 4 P's of safe sedation

The key considerations can be described as the 4 Ps of safe sedation practice, i.e. Patients, Procedure, Provider, Place.

**Patient:** Is the patient suitable? Does he/she understand (informed consent)?

**Procedure:** Can it be done safely under sedation or is general anaesthesia required?

**Provider:** Does the provider have the necessary training and skills to safely provide sedation?

**Place:** Is the place equipped? Is there a backup if things go wrong?

# Patient

It is important to recognise that not all patients undergoing minor surgical procedures need sedation; detailed explanation of the procedure and reassurance may be all that is required in most patients. Sedation may be indicated where the benefits outweigh the risks and if the provision of sedation is likely to increase the success of the procedure; for example, in anxious patients, prolonged procedures or in uncomfortable and painful procedures. Contraindications are given in Table 15.1.

## How should the patient be prepared prior to sedation and analgesia?

**1 Preoperative assessment**

A focused history, physical examination and laboratory investigations where indicated are done to identify any organ system derangements that may influence the suitability for sedation, the choice of drug and dosing and the patient's response. The patient is then categorised into ASA physical status grades I–V (Table 15.2). Patients with ASA grades I–III are suitable for sedation, but a higher degree of vigilance is required in patients with an ASA grade III and greater.

**2 Airway assessment**

Assess for a difficult airway (Table 15.3) and Mallampati classification (Table 15.4); patients with a difficult airway may not be suitable for sedation.

**3 Fasting status**

Patients are fasted according to the RCN preoperative fasting guidelines (Table 15.5). Patients should be advised if any specific medication needs to be discontinued.

**4 Informed consent**

Risks, benefits and alternative techniques should be explained and documented.

## What is the preoperative ASA physical status grading?

The American Society of Anesthesiology (ASA) physical status grading classifies patients based on the presence and severity of medical comorbidities. An 'E' is added after the grade to denote emergency surgery.

# Procedure

Commonly performed procedures in which sedation is used are dental procedures, minor surgical procedures, endoscopy, diagnostic imaging / interventional radiology, pain management and cardiology procedures.

# Provider

The medical practitioner should have the necessary training:

1 Pre-procedural assessment and optimisation
2 Proficient with monitoring techniques and equipment
3 Knowledge of the pharmacology of administered drugs and their interactions

**4** Monitoring patient's depth of sedation and cardiorespiratory function

**5** Airway management and resuscitation skills. Consider if you need anaesthetic involvement and ask early if so.

## Place

### What are the facilities required?

**1** Adequate space and lighting.

**2** Oxygen and equipment for oxygen delivery (face mask, nasal prongs, Ambu bag, C circuit).

**3** Airway equipment (oral/nasal airways, endotracheal tubes, LMA, laryngoscope).

**4** Suction apparatus.

**5** Monitoring: non-invasive blood pressure (NIBP), pulse oximetry saturation (SpO2), electrocardiogram (ECG) and end-tidal carbon dioxide ( $EtCO_2$).

**6** Drugs: sedatives, opioid analgesics, opioid and benzodiazepine antagonists and drugs for resuscitation (adrenaline, amiodarone, atropine, ephedrine).

**7** Resuscitation trolley should be in an accessible place in case of an emergency. The trolley should have a defibrillator, airway equipment, resuscitation drugs, fluids, IV cannulas and syringes.

### How to conduct sedation and analgesia for a minor surgical procedure?

After obtaining written informed consent establish intravenous access. Commence standard ASA recommended monitoring (NIBP, ECG, SpO2 and $EtCO_2$) if sedation is being used.

- Induction of sedation and analgesia: titrate dose to desirable effect.
- Maintenance of sedation: incremental doses as required.
- Monitor patient's sedation levels and cardiorespiratory status.
- Post-procedure: continue monitoring of sedation and cardiorespiratory status. Discharge when criteria met.

### Medications used

A variety of sedatives have been described for use in minor surgery including benzodiazepines, propofol and ketamine, along with opiate analgesics. If the sedation is performed by the surgeon themselves, benzodiazepines with or without opioids are commonly used. Benzodiazepines can be reversed by administration of flumazenil, while opioids can be reversed by naloxone. Reversal agents should not be used routinely, rather are used to reverse significant oversedation. Other sedatives such as propofol can cause rapid changes in level of sedation and there is no specific antidote and therefore are not safe for administration by surgeons, but rather will require anaesthetic expertise.

## Monitoring the level of sedation

Modified Ramsay score (Table 15.6) is a widely used sedation score; a sedation score of 2 or 3 is desirable. A sedation score of 4 may be acceptable if the patient can maintain their airway and has a stable cardiorespiratory status.

## Complications of sedation

**1** Respiratory system: hypoventilation, hypoxia, hypercarbia, respiratory depression and death.

**2** Cardiovascular system: hypotension and cardiovascular instability.

**3** Central nervous system: excessive sedation and anaesthesia, loss of protective airway reflexes, paradoxical response to sedation, i.e. excitation.

**4** Other – nausea, vomiting and aspiration.

## Reversal of sedation (if required)

**1** Stop further administration of sedation.

**2** Administer 100% oxygen via a re-breather mask.

**3** Clear the airway if secretions present.

**4** Support the airway if obstructed; assist ventilation if required.

**5** Administer appropriate reversal agent, use caution as reversal agents have a shorter half-life compared to the drug and a second interval dose of the sedative may be required.

**6** Call for help or anaesthetic support if appropriate.

## Discharge

There are a number of discharge criteria and scoring systems with some tailored for specific procedures. In general it is essential to ensure that:

**1** The patient is alert and oriented

**2** Sufficient time has elapsed since administration of the sedative and/or reversal agent so as to avoid re-sedation

**3** Pain is well controlled and not expected to require strong analgesics on discharge

**4** Nausea and vomiting, if present, is treated

**5** Vitals are stable and not expected to deteriorate

**6** The procedure undertaken doesn't require further postoperative monitoring for complications.

### What are the post-discharge instructions?

**1** Written and verbal information about the diet, medications, activity and follow-up.

**2** Discharge to the care of a responsible adult.

**3** Contact information in case of an emergency.

### Further reading

http://www.rcoa.ac.uk/system/files/PROPOFOL-ERCP-2014_0.pdf (accessed 20 June 2016)

https://www2.rcn.org.uk/__data/assets/pdf_file/0009/78678/002800.pdf (accessed 20 June 2016)

Safe Sedation Practice for Healthcare Procedures: Standards and Guidance. AoMRC, London 2013 (www.rcoa.ac.uk/node/15182)

# 16 General and regional anaesthesia

### Figure 16.1 Digital nerve block

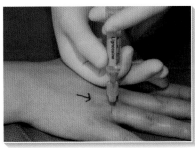

Digital nerve block at the proximal phalanx. Local anaesthetic is injected at the dorsal aspect of the hand in close proximity to the dorsal nerve. The 25G needle is then advanced towards the palmar side and further LA injected in close proximity to the palmar nerve. The procedure is repeated on the other side of the marked finger.

### Figure 16.2 Spinal anaesthesia

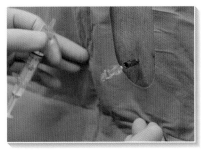

**(a)** Clear CSF flows via the 25G spinal needle from the sub arachnoid space prior to LA injection

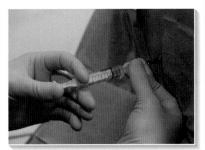

**(b)** LA injection into the subarachnoid space

### Figure 16.3 Ulnar nerve block

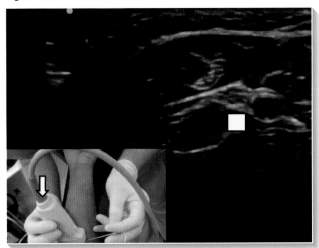

Ultrasound-guided peripheral nerve block of the ulnar nerve.
Note the ulnar nerve (above white square) lies just medial to the ulnar artery.

### Figure 16.4 Radial nerve block

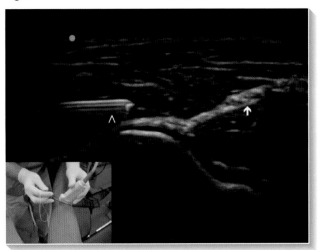

Ultrasound-guided peripheral nerve block of the radial nerve.
The needle (∧) is inserted towards the radial nerve (arrow).

*Minor Surgery at a Glance*, First Edition. Edited by Helen Mohan and Desmond Winter. © 2017 John Wiley & Sons, Ltd. Published 2017 by John Wiley & Sons, Ltd.

# Introduction

For most minor surgical procedures infiltration of local anaesthetic (LA) at the site of surgery will provide sufficient anaesthesia to allow surgery to take place; however, in some circumstances alternative techniques should be considered. Examples of such circumstances include: Surgical factors: operations involving body cavities, deep neck lumps, extensive area or depth, prolonged duration. Patient factors: anxiety, allergy to LA agents (rare), coagulopathy, local infection.

# General anaesthesia

General anaesthesia (GA) refers to a reversible state of unconsciousness that is deliberately induced to allow surgical procedures to take place.

This involves the administration of intravenous hypnotic drugs, usually in combination with opioid analgesics, with or without the addition of muscle relaxants. This form of anaesthesia must only be undertaken by appropriately trained individuals in the presence of recommended equipment and support to ensure safe practice. Once anaesthetised, the patient will usually require insertion of an airway management device, typically a laryngeal mask airway (LMA) or an endotracheal tube (ETT). These devices allow ventilation to be controlled, while also allowing the administration of anaesthetic gases to maintain the anaesthetised state until surgery has finished.

Remember when listing a patient for a procedure under GA they will need to **fast** in accordance with local guidelines, see Table 15.5 in Chapter 15. Check your local hospital policy for procedures under GA – many hospitals have a **preassessment clinic** where these patients should be reviewed prior to their admission for surgery.

# Regional anaesthesia

Regional anaesthesia refers to the administration of local anaesthetic agents in close proximity to a sensory nerve (or collection of nerves) to produce numbness in the tissues supplied by that nerve. Such techniques include central neuraxial blocks (spinal and epidural anaesthesia) and peripheral nerve blocks. They minimise the amount of LA required, thus reducing the risk of LA toxicity, and may cause less patient discomfort than high-volume LA infiltration techniques.

These techniques should also only be undertaken by an appropriately trained individual.

Selecting an appropriate technique depends on a thorough knowledge of the relevant anatomy. With any regional anaesthetic technique there is a small risk of nerve injury. This can be minimised by avoiding injection in the presence of pain or paraesthesiae on needle insertion. An aseptic technique should always be used to avoid infectious complications.

# Spinal anaesthesia

Using a spinal needle, 2–3 mL LA is placed in the subarachnoid space below the level of termination of the spinal cord (L1–L2). Injection of LA at this level will result in anaesthesia of the lower limbs and trunk. The 'height' of the block will be influenced by the amount of LA injected. This type of anaesthetic is commonly used for orthopaedic procedures of the lower limbs and for lower abdominal surgery.

# Epidural anaesthesia

This technique involves the placement of a catheter in the epidural space, which contains the spinal nerve roots as they emerge from the spinal cord. LA can then be delivered to the space to provide effective analgesia. This technique is generally reserved for conditions that require ongoing analgesia over an extended period e.g. labour.

## Pre- and post-op considerations

Remember for both spinal and epidural anaesthesia, low molecular weight heparin and other anticoagulants must be held preoperatively and for a duration post-operatively – check local guidelines. Also, make sure patients have passed urine and are not in urinary retention prior to discharge.

# Peripheral nerve blocks

Peripheral nerve blocks can facilitate surgery in the head and neck and in the peripheries. For these blocks, as little as 1 or 2 mL of LA may be sufficient to produce the desired effect, although this will depend on the proximity of the needle tip to the nerve and the size of the sensory nerve.

Ultrasound is often used to facilitate correct anatomical identification. Make sure to document neurovascular status prior to peripheral nerve blocks, particularly in trauma.

## Head and neck

The supraorbital and supratrochlear nerves can be blocked by the infiltration of 5–7 mL of LA along the lower border of the medial two-thirds of the eyebrow. This will produce anaesthesia of the forehead. The infraorbital nerve supplies the upper lip, cheek and part of the nose, and can be blocked as it emerges at the infraorbital foramen on the lower border of the orbit. The mental nerve can be blocked as it emerges from the mental foramen, and it supplies sensation to the lower lip and chin.

The superficial cervical plexus can be blocked by infiltrating LA along the posterior border of sternocleidomastoid muscle. This produces numbness of the superficial structures of the posterior head, neck and shoulder.

## Upper limb

The radial nerve supplies sensation to the radial half of the dorsum of the hand, the back of the thumb, and part of the dorsum of the index finger. It can be blocked at the wrist by injecting 3 mL of LA just lateral to the radial artery, then infiltrating LA subcutaneously along the proximal border of the anatomical snuffbox to the middle of the posterior aspect of the wrist.

The ulnar nerve supplies sensation to the ulnar side of the palm and to the ulnar half of the dorsum of the hand, little finger and ulnar side of the ring finger. It can be blocked by injecting 5–7 mL LA deep to the tendon of flexor carpi ulnaris and subcutaneous infiltration of 3–4 mL LA from the ulnar styloid on the dorsal surface of the wrist.

The median nerve supplies sensation to the lateral surface of the palm, the flexor aspect of the thumb, index finger, middle finger and radial side of the ring finger. It can be blocked at the skin crease of the wrist by insertion of a needle between the tendons of flexor carpi radialis and palmaris longus. The needle is advanced at 45° until a loss of resistance is felt as the needle passes through the flexor retinaculum; 2–5 mL LA are injected to block the nerve. Subcutaneous infiltration of a further 0.5–1.0 mL above the retinaculum will block the superficial palmar branch.

Digital nerves supply sensation to the fingers. They can be blocked by the injection of 3–5 mL LA adjacent to the proximal phalanx on both sides. Alternatively, they can be blocked adjacent to the metacarpal head. *Adrenaline containing solutions are not recommended for use in extremities as they may lead to ischaemia.*

## Lower limb

The femoral nerve is derived from the L2 to L4 nerve roots via the lumbar plexus. It supplies sensation to the anterior and medial thigh and knee joint. It emerges beneath the inguinal ligament lateral to the femoral artery and vein, where it can be blocked using appropriate nerve localisation techniques (ultrasound guidance or peripheral nerve stimulation) to minimise the risks of intraneural injection.

The femoral nerve terminates as the saphenous nerve, which divides into superficial branches over the flat surface of the tibia on the anteromedial aspect of the leg. It supplies sensation to a variable territory over the medial leg, ankle and foot. The saphenous nerve can be blocked by subcutaneous infiltration of 5–10 mL of LA along the flat surface of the tibia.

The sciatic nerve is derived from the ventral rami of L4–S3 via the sacral plexus, and passes through the greater sciatic foramen of the pelvis to run along the posterior thigh. It divides into the common peroneal nerve and the tibial nerve above the knee. The sciatic nerve may be blocked by one of a number of described techniques along its course in the thigh.

The common peroneal nerve passes around the neck of the fibula, where it is very superficial, and continues along the anterolateral compartment of the leg. It divides into superficial and deep peroneal nerves at the ankle.

The superficial peroneal nerve can be blocked by subcutaneous infiltration of LA along the dorsum of the foot between the medial and lateral malleoli. This nerve supplies sensation to the dorsum of the foot aside from the first interdigital cleft. The **deep** peroneal nerve can be blocked by injection of 3–5 mL of LA lateral to the dorsalis pedis artery. This anaesthetises the skin between the first and second toes.

The tibial nerve runs in the posterior compartment of the leg, and divides into the posterior tibial and sural nerves. The posterior tibial nerve can be blocked by the injection of 5–10 mL of LA at the midpoint between the medial malleolus and the heel, posterolateral to the posterior tibial artery. This will provide anaesthesia to the heel, plantar portion of the toes, and the sole of the foot.

The sural nerve supplies sensation to the lateral part of the foot and the lateral proximal aspect of the sole of the foot. It can be blocked by subcutaneous infiltration of 5–10 mL LA between the lateral malleolus and the calcaneal tendon.

Digital nerve blocks can be performed to facilitate surgery on ingrown toenails by injection of 3–5 mL of LA on either side of the proximal phalanx. Adrenaline-containing solutions are not recommended for use in extremities as they may lead to ischaemia.

### Further reading

Harmon D. *Peripheral Nerve Blocks & Peri-operative Pain Relief.* Philadelphia: Saunders/Elsevier; 2011.

Miller's Anesthesia. 7th edn. Philadelphia, PA: Churchill Livingstone/Elsevier; 2010.

Salam GA. Regional anesthesia for office procedures: Part I. Head and neck surgeries. *American Family Physician* 2004 Feb 1;69(3):585–90.

Salam GA. Regional anesthesia for office procedures: Part II. Extremity and inguinal area surgeries. *American Family Physician* 2004; 69 (4): 896–900.

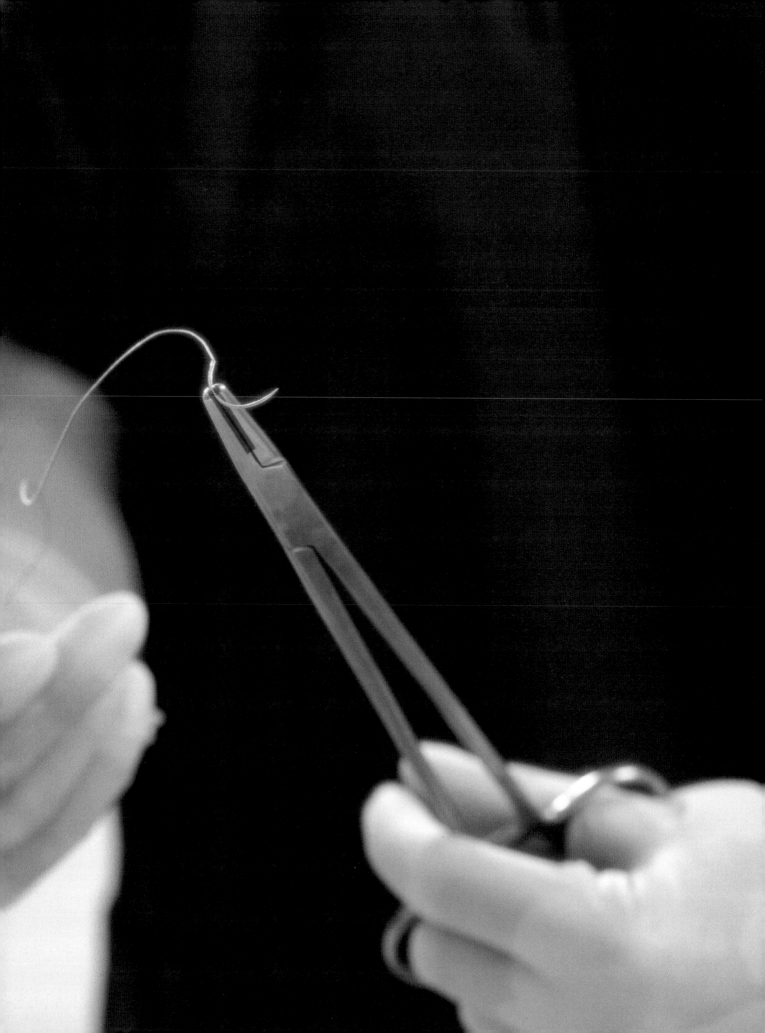

# Core surgical knowledge

Part 3

## Chapters

# 17 Skin incisions

**Figure 17.1**  Scalpel blades

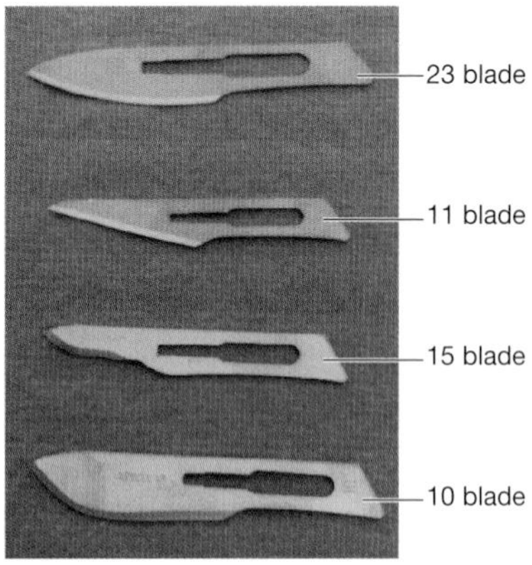

23 blade

11 blade

15 blade

10 blade

**(a)**

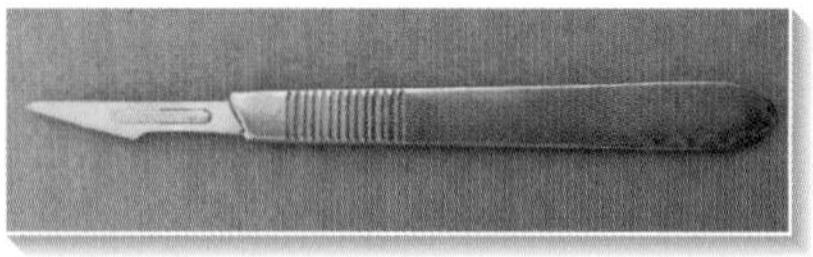

**(b)**  Scalpel with 11 blade

**Figure 17.2**  Holding a scalpel

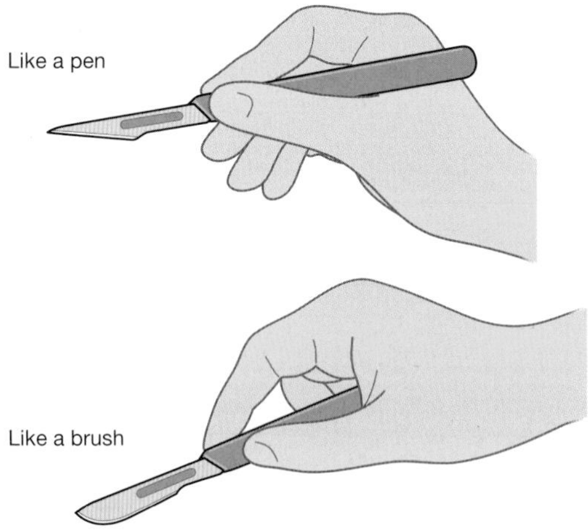

Like a pen

Like a brush

**Figure 17.3**  Incisions

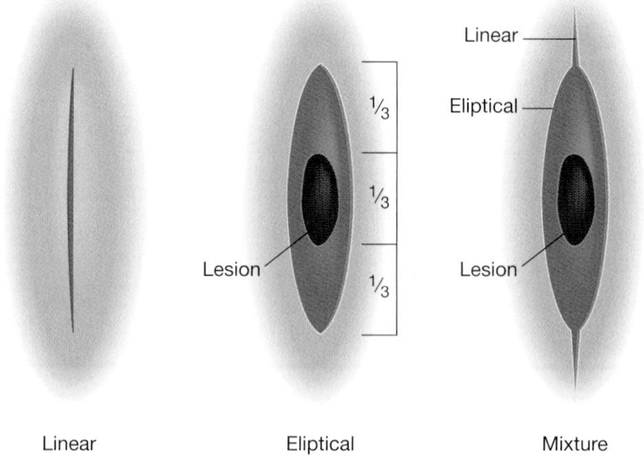

Linear

Eliptical

Lesion

Linear

1/3

1/3

1/3

Lesion

Eliptical

Lesion

Mixture

**Figure 17.4**  Langer's lines

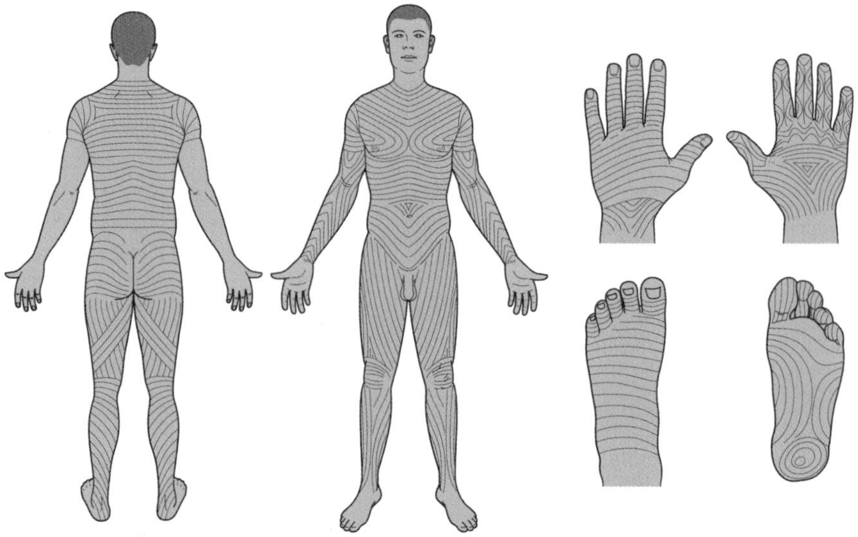

*Minor Surgery at a Glance*, First Edition. Edited by Helen Mohan and Desmond Winter. © 2017 John Wiley & Sons, Ltd. Published 2017 by John Wiley & Sons, Ltd.

# Scalpels

Scalpels can have a reusable handle with a disposable blade, or the entire blade and handle may be integrated and disposable. For reusable handles, the blade is grasped firmly on the non-sharpened edge with a needle holder and the centre of the handle is placed in the hole in the blade and gently slid on. Exercise extreme caution when mounting a blade that it does not snap off and injure you or your assistants.

In general, there are four different size blades commonly used (Figure 17.1).

**15 Blade:** This has a small curved cutting edge. It is useful for performing precise skin incisions.

**11 Blade:** This is a triangular long blade and its most common use is stab incisions, for example, laparoscopic port sites, drainage of an abscess, shave biopsy.

**10 or 23 Blade:** These have a large cutting surface for long incisions.

# Holding the scalpel to make an incision

**Stab incisions (11 Blade):** For stab incisions, hold the scalpel like a pen.

**Linear incisions:** For linear incisions, hold the scalpel like a brush or violin bow (Figure 17.2).

# Basic principles for incision

**1 Accessibility.** The incision should provide direct anatomical access while providing room for manoeuvre. The incision must be maximally utilised to facilitate exposure. This can be aided with the use of gentle retraction, positioning and illumination.
**2 Extensibility.** If the original incision is inadequate, there must be anticipation of extension to facilitate greater exposure and accessibility, without causing extensive damage.
**3 Tension-free closure.** Wound closure must meet the requirements of good approximation, healthy edges, and be tension free to provide optimal wound integrity.

When making an incision for excising a suspected malignant skin lesion, be careful not to saucerise the wound (i.e. do not creep inwards with the deep margin), and cut down far enough into the dermis.

# Minor surgical incisions

See Figure 17.3 for common incisions in minor surgery. In general, linear incisions are used for lipomata and occasionally for foreign bodies, while elliptical incisions are used for skin lesions and sebaceous cysts. In cosmetically sensitive areas, adaptations may be used, for example, an elliptical incision with linear extension at either end (Figure 17.3) When performing an elliptical excision, the length of the ellipse should be at least three times its width to prevent 'dog ears'. Adaptations may be used in cosmetically sensitive areas (e.g. linear extension of an ellipse; Figure 17.3).

# Techniques for a good scar

**1** Develop meticulous tissue handling skills.
**2** Respect the relaxed skin tension lines (RSTLs) and lines of maximal extensibility (LMEs). Langer's lines were traditionally used to guide the optimum lines for incision, and are based on cadaveric studies. (See Figure 17.4 for a diagram of Langer's lines.) A more modern concept described by Borges are RSTLs, which are now generally used instead. (See Chapter 18 for Langer's lines on face.) Incisions made parallel to Langer's or RSTLs are associated with improved healing. Remember that they apply to the trunk and limbs, not just the head and neck.
**3** Use toothed forceps when handling skin edges to preserve them.
**4** Be vigilant for hair strands entering the wound margin (best avoided).

# Electrodissection to incise

The other option to using a scalpel to make an incision, is to use cutting diathermy. Often, the initial breach of the skin is performed with a scalpel, followed by diathermy for the deeper layers, but using cutting diathermy is also an accepted technique for larger lesions. Follow the principles described in the Chapter 21 on diathermy.

# 18 Principles of wound closure

**Figure 18.1** Relaxed skin tension lines of the face

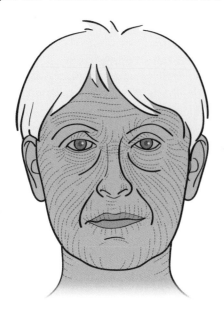

**Figure 18.2** Using Langer's lines to determine orientation of incisions

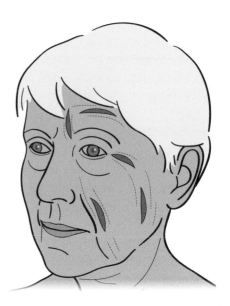

**Figure 18.3** Suturing of the skin
The placement of a dermal suture will aid in approximation of the tissue to reduce the tension on the wound. A superficial suture is placed to accurately approximate the edges, and the aim of this suture is to evert the skin edges

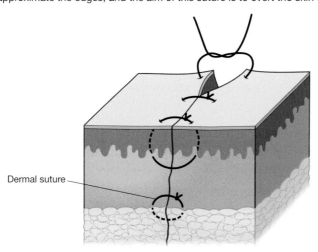

Dermal suture

## Plan the skin incision

Planning the surgical procedure will help ensure the best outcome for the patient. In the elective setting, the aim is to achieve a cosmetically pleasing fine line scar, especially on exposed areas of the body, such as the face.

It is very useful to mark the outline of the skin lesion and the planned skin incision *prior* to injection of local anaesthetic as it may distort anatomy.

## Obtaining a fine line scar

There are two important technical factors to consider when trying to achieve a fine line scar.

**1** The orientation of the final scar should lie in the same direction as the relaxed skin tension lines (or 'Langer's lines'), which are similar to wrinkle lines (Figure 18.1). This is especially important on the face (Figure 18.2).

*Minor Surgery at a Glance*, First Edition. Edited by Helen Mohan and Desmond Winter. © 2017 John Wiley & Sons, Ltd. Published 2017 by John Wiley & Sons, Ltd.

**2** The wound edges should be approximated and slightly everted (Figure 18.3), because as the wound matures, the scar tends to widen.

## Choosing the suture size

Sutures range in size from 00 (very large, not for minor surgery) to 11-0 (used for microvascular anastomosis). Generally, sizes varying from 3-0 to 5-0 are used in minor surgery.

On the face, it is best to use small sutures, like 5-0 or 6-0. For other areas, a 4-0 suture achieves the right balance between strength and cosmesis. A 3-0 suture may be ideal for large wounds on the back where wound tension can be high.

## Choosing the suture material

| Material | Trade name | Types | Strength | Indications |
|---|---|---|---|---|
| **Absorbable** | | | | |
| Poliglecaprone 25 Glycolmer 631 | Monocryl Biosyn | Synthetic monofilament | Half-life 14 days. Completely absorbed 91–119 days | Deep dermal and subcuticular sutures |
| Glycolide/ Lactide co-polymer | Vicryl Polysorb | Synthetic braided | Holds its tensile strength for 3–4 weeks. Completely absorbed within 60 days | Vessel ligation. Soft tissue approximation |
| **Non-absorbable** | | | | |
| Nylon | Ethilon Monosof | Monofilament | Loses 20% suture strength per year | Skin sutures |
| Polypropylene | Prolene Surgipro | Monofilament | Non-absorbable | Skin sutures |

## Suture placement

**Face:** Sutures should be approximately 2–3 mm from the skin edge and 3–5 mm apart.

**Elsewhere on the body:** Sutures should be approximately 3–4 mm from the skin edge and 5–10 mm apart. Always start on the corner furthest away and work towards yourself.

## Technique for simple interrupted sutures

To ensure that the edges evert, the needle tip should enter at a 90 degree angle to the skin. Turn your wrist gently to drive the needle through the skin layers. Start from the outside, go through the epidermis and into the subcutaneous tissue on one side. Then remount the needle to enter the subcutaneous tissue on the opposite side, and come out the epidermis. Tie the suture to one side of the wound. (See Figure 18.3.)

## When should I use a different suturing technique?

**1** Simple (interrupted/continuous): Easiest option. Used for most skin suturing. Continuous can be used to help reduce bleeding from the skin edges (especially with scalp lacerations).
**2** Mattress sutures (horizontal/vertical): Used when it is more challenging to evert the skin edges.
**3** Buried intradermal or subcutaneous sutures: Useful for gaping wounds to reduce tension on wound closure.

### Is stapling a suitable option?

Skin stapling is a quicker option than suturing and is commonly employed in large wounds (e.g. on the leg) or in areas where it is necessary to minimise blood loss from the wound (e.g. scalp).

It is important to avoid placing staples on the face as they can cause significant scarring.

When placing staples, it is very important to approximate and evert the skin edges using forceps. Staples are usually placed 1 cm apart.

### Skin adhesives

These may be used for small lacerations. They are very useful in paediatrics. The skin should be approximated and then a layer of tissue adhesive applied until it has set. It is important to remember that wound irrigation and debridement may be necessary before applying tissue adhesive. Tissue adhesives have the advantage of absorbing within a week usually. Do not use in conjunction with ointments as they may dissolve the adhesive.

### Adhesive tapes

These can be useful in small wounds to bring the skin edges together, or following suture removal, to provide extra strength to the wound.

They are particularly useful in children. They should not be used where there is excessive tension on the skin edges.

## Removing sutures

Face: 5 days
Hand: 10–14 days
Limbs/Back: 10–14 days

## Anaesthesia

For details of local anaesthetic technique, see chapter 15 Local Anaesthesia.

# 19 Sutures

**Figure 19.1** Interpreting a suture packet

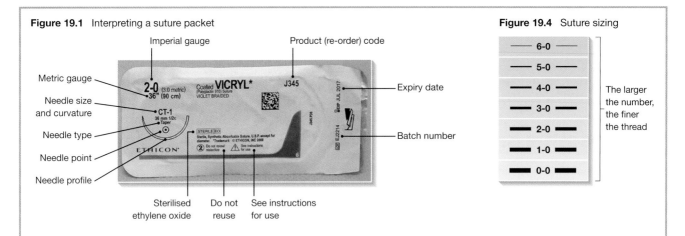

Metric gauge

Needle size and curvature

Needle type

Needle point

Needle profile

Imperial gauge

Product (re-order) code

2-0 (3.0 metric)
36" (90 cm)

CT-1
36 mm 1/2c
Taper

Coated VICRYL*
Polyglactin 910 Suture
VIOLET BRAIDED

J345

Expiry date

Batch number

Sterilised ethylene oxide

Do not reuse

See instructions for use

**Figure 19.4** Suture sizing

6-0
5-0
4-0
3-0
2-0
1-0
0-0

The larger the number, the finer the thread

**Figure 19.2** Suture materials

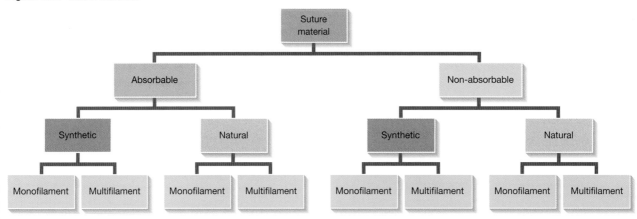

Suture material

Absorbable — Non-absorbable

Absorbable: Synthetic, Natural
Non-absorbable: Synthetic, Natural

Synthetic (Absorbable): Monofilament, Multifilament
Natural (Absorbable): Monofilament, Multifilament
Synthetic (Non-absorbable): Monofilament, Multifilament
Natural (Non-absorbable): Monofilament, Multifilament

**Figure 19.3** Overview of some commonly used suture materials and their uses

| | Suture | Material | Source | Monofilament/Braided | Properties |
|---|---|---|---|---|---|
| **Absorbable** | Catgut | Purified animal intestine | Natural | Monofilament | • Marked inflammatory response<br>• Absorbed by proteolytic digestion<br>• Not used in UK |
| | Monocryl | Polyglecaprone 25 | Synthetic | Monofilament | • Used for subcuticular closure |
| | Vicryl | Polyglactin 910 | Synthetic | Braided | • Handles well |
| | Vicryl rapide | Polyglactin 910 | Synthetic | Braided | • Rapid absorption |
| | PDS II | Polydioxanone | Synthetic | Monofilament | • Slow absorption |
| **Non-absorbable** | Silk | Natural silk | Natural | Braided | • Handles well<br>• Marked inflammatory reaction<br>• Degrades without absorption<br>• Not for skin closure |
| | Mersilene | Polyester | Synthetic | Braided/monofilament | • High tensile strength |
| | Ethilon | Nylon-polyamide | Synthetic | Monofilament | • Minimal tissue reaction |
| | Prolene | Polypropylene | Synthetic | Monofilament | • Characteristic blue thread |

*Minor Surgery at a Glance*, First Edition. Edited by Helen Mohan and Desmond Winter. © 2017 John Wiley & Sons, Ltd. Published 2017 by John Wiley & Sons, Ltd.

# Introduction

The purpose of a suture material is to hold a wound in adequate apposition until such time that the natural healing process is sufficiently well established. The earliest evidence of the use of sutures can be traced to ancient times where materials such as linen and wool threads were used to close wounds. Technological advances made in suture and needle technology allowed for the development of more sophisticated sutures e.g. nylon and polyester in the 1930s and synthetic polymer fibres e.g. polyglycolic acid and polyglactic acid in the 1960s. These alternatives have largely superseded catgut in the developed world.

# Properties of the ideal suture material

- Good handling characteristics
- No tissue reaction
- Adequate tensile strength
- Sterile
- Non-electrolytic
- Non-allergenic
- Inexpensive.

# Types of suture material

Suture materials are broadly classified as being absorbable or non-absorbable. They can be further subcategorised into braided (multifilament) or non-braided (monofilament) (Figures 19.1, 19.2 and 19.3).

## Non-absorbable sutures

Non-absorbable sutures remain in place until they are removed. Because the body does not dissolve them, they are less tissue-reactive and therefore leave less scarring as long as they are removed in a timely fashion. The various parts of the body heal at different speeds. Typically, sutures used on the face are removed by 5 days, scalp wounds 7–10 days, limbs 10–14 days, joints 14 days and trunk of the body 10–14 days.

## Absorbable sutures

Absorbable sutures are dissolved by the body and as such do not need to be removed. However, absorbable sutures tend to leave a more pronounced scar when used as skin sutures. Absorbable sutures are primarily used within the subcutaneous layer of skin, where they are well hidden. It is sometimes difficult to get patients to return for suture removal. If this is a concern, an absorbable suture should be used for skin closure. The patient should be forewarned that absorbable sutures will probably result in a more noticeable scar than non-absorbable sutures when removed. As it is often difficult to remove stitches from children, absorbable materials may be used when suturing their wounds.

Much variation exists on the rate of absorption, which depends greatly on the breaking strength of the knotted fibre. This translates into a specific number of days and an approximate percentage of tensile strength remaining. For example, for polyglactin 910 (Vicryl Rapide), it may be as little as 5 days/50%.

## Braided sutures

Braided sutures are comprised of several thin strands of the suture material twisted together. Braided sutures are easier to tie than non-braided sutures. However, braided sutures have little interstices in the suture material, which can be a place for bacteria to lurk.

## Non-braided sutures

Non-braided sutures are simply a monofilament, a single strand. They are not made up of the little subunits found in a braided suture. Non-braided sutures are recommended for most skin closure, especially wounds that may be at risk for infection.

# Suture sizes

Sutures are sized by the United States Pharmacopoeia (USP) scale (Figure 19.4). The larger the number, the smaller the size of the suture. Sizes 3-0 and 6-0 are most commonly used. It is best to use small sutures on the face, such as 5-0 or 6-0. Smaller sutures are associated with less scarring. On areas where cosmetic concerns are less important, 3-0 or 4-0 sutures are best because the thicker sutures are stronger. As well as superficial sutures, thicker tissues (e.g. trunk) often need subcutaneous absorbable closure too.

**Table 19.2** Suture indications for superficial closure by location

| | |
|---|---|
| Scalp, torso (chest, back, abdomen), extremities | Superficial non-absorbable suture: 4-0 or 5-0 |
| Face, eyebrow, nose, lip | Superficial non-absorbable suture: 6-0 |
| Ear, eyelid | Superficial non-absorbable suture: 6-0 |
| Hand | Superficial non-absorbable suture: 5-0 |
| Foot or sole | Superficial non-absorbable suture: 3-0 or 4-0 |

### Further reading

Jain SK, Stoker DL, Tanwar R. *Basic Surgical Skills and Techniques.* Jaypee Brothers, Medical Publishers Pvt Limited; 2013.

Practical Plastic Surgery for Nonsurgeons. Chapter 1: Suturing The Basics. http://practicalplasticsurgery.org/docs/Practical_01.pdf (accessed 24 June 2016).

Venkataram M. *Textbook on Cutaneous and Aesthetic Surgery.* Jaypee Brothers, Medical Publishers Pvt Limited; 2012.

# 20 Needles

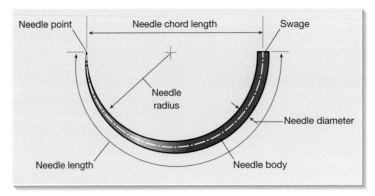

**Figure 20.1** Anatomy of a surgical needle

Needle point
Needle chord length
Swage
Needle radius
Needle diameter
Needle length
Needle body

**Figure 20.2** Needle shapes

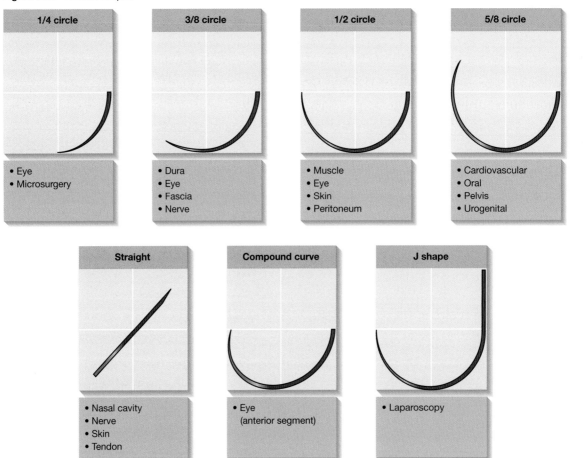

**1/4 circle**
- Eye
- Microsurgery

**3/8 circle**
- Dura
- Eye
- Fascia
- Nerve

**1/2 circle**
- Muscle
- Eye
- Skin
- Peritoneum

**5/8 circle**
- Cardiovascular
- Oral
- Pelvis
- Urogenital

**Straight**
- Nasal cavity
- Nerve
- Skin
- Tendon

**Compound curve**
- Eye (anterior segment)

**J shape**
- Laparoscopy

*Minor Surgery at a Glance,* First Edition. Edited by Helen Mohan and Desmond Winter. © 2017 John Wiley & Sons, Ltd. Published 2017 by John Wiley & Sons, Ltd.

# Understanding surgical needles

Figure 20.1 shows the anatomy of a surgical needle.

**Needle point:** Penetration of a needle is dependent on the point. Each specific point is designed and produced to the required degree of sharpness to penetrate smoothly the types of tissues to be sutured.

**Chord length:** This is the straight-line distance from the point of a curved needle to the swage. This can vary from 2 mm to more than 2 inches. Length is a determining factor in the width of bite taken by the needle.

**Swage:** This is the area in which the suture is attached to the needle. The swage area is of specific importance to the relationship of needle and suture thicknesses. It is also the weakest point of the needle. The objective of the swage area is to achieve the closest one-to-one suture needle ratio as possible. A one-to-one needle ratio reduces additional trauma that may be caused by the needle or the suture.

**Needle diameter:** The gauge or thickness of the needle wire. Needle diameter various from 30 microns to over 1 mm. The diameter equals the size of the needle track – except with spatulated or cutting designs.

**Needle radius:** If the curvature of the needle were to continue to make a full circle, the radius of the curvature is the distance from the centre of the circle to the body of the needle. Think of the needle as part of a circle.

# Selecting a needle

The two factors used in selecting a needle are size, and when a cutting or tapered needle is required. While there are exceptions, in general tapered needles are used inside the body such as on bowel, fascia or muscle where the tissue is more easily pierced. Cutting needles are used for skin and very tough tissue such as bone and tendon.

Needles are available in various shapes to accommodate the desired depth in specific tissue (Figure 20.2). Selection of the needle shape is dependent on the size and depth of the area to be sutured. Use of the ¼ circle needle is often limited to ophthalmic and microsurgical procedures. A commonly used curved needle is the ⅜ circle. These needles can be easily manipulated in relatively large and superficial wounds such as closure of the dermis. Because a large arc of manipulation is required, ⅜ circle needles can be awkward or impossible to use in deep cavities such as the pelvis or in other small difficult-to-access locations. A ½ circle needle is relatively easy to use in these confined locations, although it requires more rotation of the wrist than a ⅜ circle. The tip of a ½ circle needle can become obscured by tissue deep in the pelvic cavity for example. When this occurs the surgeon may have difficulty locating the point to reposition the needle holder and pull the needle through tissue. A ⅝ circle needle may be useful in this situation, as may a 'J' needle. Straight needles are generally used for skin and compound curved needles for ophthalmics.

# 21 Diathermy

**Figure 21.1** Electrical circuit: electrical current is pushed by the generator through a resistor producing heating

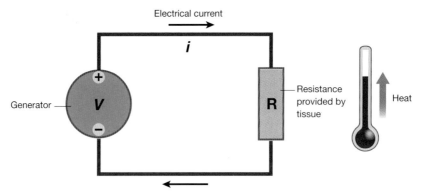

Electrical current

*i*

Generator — **V**

**R** — Resistance provided by tissue

Heat

**Figure 21.2** Monopolar and bipolar electrosurgery

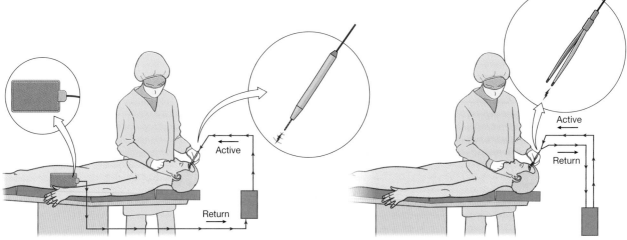

Active

Return

Active

Return

**Figure 21.3** Type of current and effects

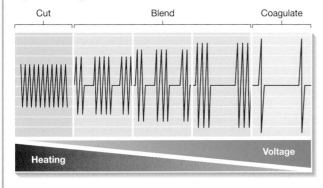

Cut    Blend    Coagulate

Heating    Voltage

**Figure 21.4** Cut and coagulate

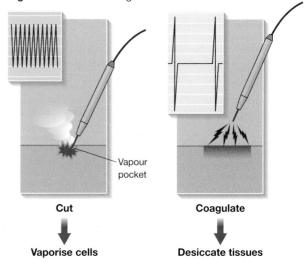

Vapour pocket

**Cut**

↓

**Vaporise cells**

**Coagulate**

↓

**Desiccate tissues**

*Minor Surgery at a Glance*, First Edition. Edited by Helen Mohan and Desmond Winter. © 2017 John Wiley & Sons, Ltd. Published 2017 by John Wiley & Sons, Ltd.

# Introduction

Electrosurgical tools use specific waveforms of high-frequency electrical current to coagulate and cut tissues. Nowadays diathermy (or 'Bovie' after William Bovie who developed the first commercially available generator) is a fundamental instrument in all types of surgery. The surgeon should be familiar with the principles of electrosurgery and potential complications.

## Definitions

**Diathermy:** (from the Greek word for "heating through") electrical induced heat.

**Cautery:** is a device or substance used to destroy tissue for medical reasons.

**Electrocautery:** device able to destroy tissues using diathermy.

**Electrosurgery:** is the application of an electric current to incise, coagulate or dry tissue.

# Principles in electrosurgery

An electrosurgical generator is a device which has the ability to create a force that conducts a flow of electrons ($I$) through a resistance ($R$) following Ohm's law $I = V/R$ where $V$ is the potential difference ($V$) created by the generator. (Figure 21.1) Biological tissues provide the resistance ($R$). According to Joule's first law, the heat ($Q$) is produced by a resistance traversed by an electrical current $Q = I^2 \times R = V^2/R$. To reduce neuromuscular stimulation and avoid electrocution, electrosurgery is performed with an alternating current (AC) at frequencies between 200 kHz and 3 MHz (below 100 kHz electrical current stimulate nerve and muscles). Modern generators are able to produce various waveforms and frequencies resulting in a variety of effect on tissues.

# Types of diathermy

**Monopolar:** The electrical current flows through two remote electrodes and the patient body forms a major element of the electrical circuit. (Figure 21.2) The active electrode corresponds to a tip of a special pencil in the hand of the surgeon. The return electrode is a large electrical plate connected somewhere on the patient's skin. The current density increase at the tip of the smaller electrode resulting in an increased heating effect and is rapidly dissipates with distance. Active electrodes are available in a variety of tips.

*Advantages:* Allows a fast and effective coagulation/cut effect.

**Bipolar:** active output and patient return functions are both accomplished at the site of surgery. Current path is confined to tissue grasped between two forceps tines with similar size.

*Advantages:*
- Electrical current pass only through the tissue grasped
- Less heating effect of the surrounding tissue
- More precise.

# Tissue effects

**Cut:** A constant AC current waveform (voltage: 500–1000 V) is used to produce an extremely rapid heating (> 400°C) resulting in the vaporisation of cells. The vapour pocket created on the tip of the electrodes slides through tissues producing a precise incision (Figure 21.3).

**Coagulate:** Interrupted pulses of current (high voltage up to 6000 V, 50–100 Hz) are used to desiccate tissues. Because of a slower heating time, the vapour pocket is not created. Less power is delivered and the cells are destroyed in the point of contact with the tip. Consequently, the small vessels are sealed and haemostasis achieved (Figure 21.4).

**Blended current:** A mixture of pulsed and continuous waveform (current is applied for up to 50% of the time and at voltages of up to 2000 V) is used to produce a simultaneous cut and coagulate effect.

**Fulguration:** The active electrode is kept at a distance from the tissue. High voltage is needed to drive the current through the resistance of air. An electrical arc is generated. The resistance of the fulgurated tissue increases and the current shifts to adjacent area with less resistance.

# Using diathermy

**Pre-operative considerations**
- Remove body piercing and jewellery.
- Decide on monopolar versus bipolar.
- Check that the return electrode (plate) is well fixed on clean and shaved skin, as close as possible to the wound.
- Avoid placing the return electrodes over bony protuberances, metallic implants, scar tissue or ECG electrodes.
- Check that the generator is set up according to the manufacturers' recommended settings based on the procedure performed.

**Perioperative considerations**
- The initial skin incision can be made using a scalpel blade and then the deep tissues divided using diathermy. Alternatively, some prefer the use of cutting diathermy for incising the skin. A systematic review has shown no difference in wound complication rates between these two approaches.
- The tip of the pencil should be held slightly away from tissues for cutting.
- Desiccation occurs when electrodes are in direct contact with the tissues.
- The longer the generator is activated, the more heat is produced and diffuses into adjacent tissues. The surgeon should be quick and move fast in order to avoid heat injuries.
- The formation of eschar leads to increased resistance. Keeping the electrodes clean will improve performance.
- The concomitant use of two electrosurgery devices on one patient is prohibited.
- Avoid relocating the return plate after it has been applied. Never cut or reduce the size of the return plate.

# Risks and complications

Accidental burns caused by:
- Inadvertent contact of activated electrode on tissues
- Direct coupling: a metallic instrument in contact with the active electrode and tissues
- Capacitive coupling
- An insulation failure of cables and electrodes
- An inadequate contact between skin and return electrode
- The combustion of alcohol skin preparation
- Electrode temperature after a prolonged use.

    Avoid monopolar electrosurgery in the presence of an implanted pacemaker.

    Also avoid monopolar electrosurgery on the digits and penis.

# 22 Dressings

**Figure 22.1** Microporous dressing (Steri-strip®)

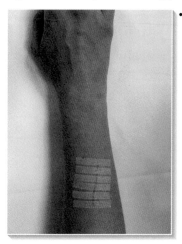

- Directly applied on the wound. This dressing may be applied perpendicular to the wound, pulling the skin edges on either together. Some surgeons apply microporous dressings, e.g. Steri-strips® parallel to the wound alternatively

**Figure 22.2** Simple dressing

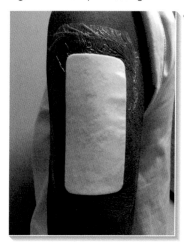

- Waterproof dressing (e.g. Opsite®, Tegaderm®) or self-adhesive breathable absorbent dressing (e.g. Mepore®)

**Figure 22.3** Absorbent dressings

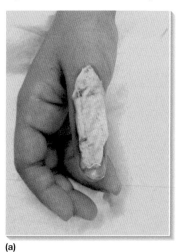

(a)

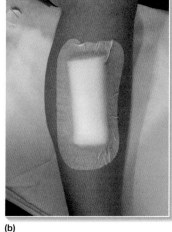

(b)

- Alginate (e.g. Kaltostat®): these dressings are seaweed derived and are useful for wounds with moderate to heavy exudate. They absorb exudate and create a gel like dressing. They can come as a ribbon or as a sheet
- Hydrofibers (e.g. Aquacel®): for heavy exudate
- Hydrocolloid dressing (e.g. DuoDERM®, Granuflex®): for wounds with a moderate exudate, like alginate dressings they absorb exudate and create a gel like dressing
- Ionic silver impregnated hydrofiber dressings may be used for colonised wounds, e.g. Aquacel Ag

**Figure 22.4** Vacuum dressings

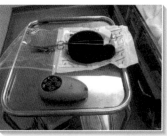

(a) VAC dressings

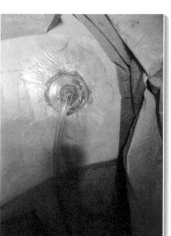

(b) VAC dressing in place

Vacuum assisted closure (VAC dressings) use foam, hydrocolloid dressings and negative pressure wound therapy

- Foam: keeps a moist environment and absorbs the exudate-excess. The foam is placed in the wound cavity
- Hydrocolloid dressing: these can be used to provide a skin barrier to protect the skin around a VAC dressing. VAC dressings may or may not include continuous wound irrigation

*Minor Surgery at a Glance*, First Edition. Edited by Helen Mohan and Desmond Winter. © 2017 John Wiley & Sons, Ltd. Published 2017 by John Wiley & Sons, Ltd.

# Choosing a dressing

## When is the dressing supposed to be changed?

• After 48–72 hours, if the dressing is not imbibed by blood, pus or exudate.

• For an uncomplicated wound, the dressing can be changed by the patient or a member of the family.

• For a complicated wound (e.g. secondary intention, heavy exudate, high risk of dehiscence) it is preferable to arrange an appointment in a dressing clinic or with a public health nurse in the community

• For pressure dressings, remove after 24–48 hours.

## When can the patient take a shower?

• Timing of showering post-operatively is controversial. With a waterproof dressing covering the surgical site, the patient can take a shower the same day as surgery.

• After 48-72 hours, the patient can take a shower without any dressing if the wound is completely dry.

• Educate the patient not to remove microporous dressings (e.g. Steri-strip®) (Figure 22.1). They will come off by themselves (usually after 7–10 days).

For wounds healing by primary intention, usually a simple dressing will suffice (Figure 22.2).

If there is an ooze of blood, a compression dressing can assist in haemostasis. Generally, these should be applied only in the presence of a slight ooze. If blood is oozing through the pressure dressing, consider whether you need to evacuate the haematoma in theatre and achieve haemostasis. Avoid pulling and damaging the skin when applying a compression dressing, and if on a limb ensure you haven't caused distal ischaemia if using a circumferential dressing.

For wounds healing by secondary intention or for infected cavities, absorbent dressings may be required to deal with wound exudate (Figure 22.3).

In cases with heavy wound exudate, VAC dressings can aid healing (Figure 22.4). Ensure the patient knows how often their dressing needs to be changed and that the dressing required is clearly communicated to the person who will be changing it.

Most hospitals will have a wound care nurse who can advise on difficult wounds and dressings.

# 23 Haemostasis

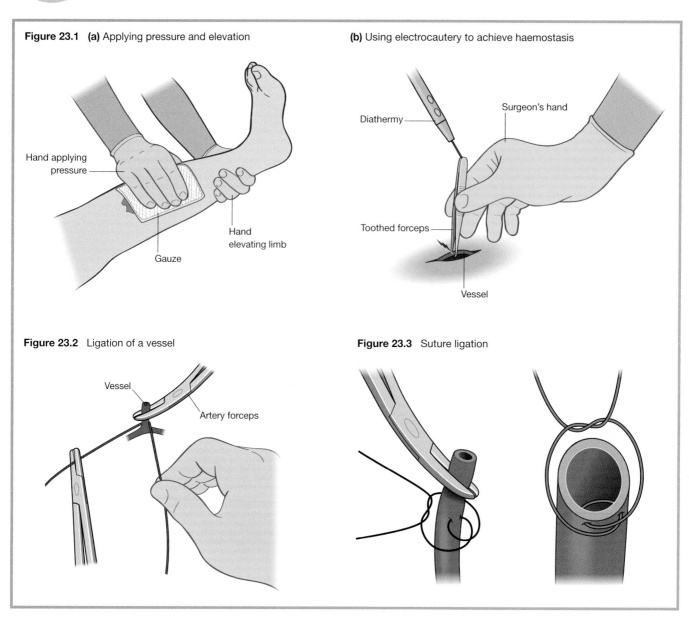

**Figure 23.1 (a)** Applying pressure and elevation

Hand applying pressure

Gauze

Hand elevating limb

**(b)** Using electrocautery to achieve haemostasis

Diathermy

Surgeon's hand

Toothed forceps

Vessel

**Figure 23.2** Ligation of a vessel

Vessel

Artery forceps

**Figure 23.3** Suture ligation

## Pressure and elevation

The easiest and simplest way to achieve haemostasis is to apply pressure and elevate the affected part if possible (Figure 23.1a). Pressure may be direct (e.g. if you visualise a bleeding arteriole during a procedure and you apply pressure with forceps), or indirect (e.g. if you compress a wound with gauze to reduce bleeding). Pressure can be applied manually, or using a compression dressing. In general, if applying pressure to a wound for haemostasis, press firmly and time using a clock for a minimum of 2 minutes.

Compression dressings can assist in haemostasis if there is a small ooze but are inappropriate for significant bleeding, and should not be an alternative to adequate primary haemostasis. Compression dressings are discussed in more detail in Chapter 22 on dressings.

For wounds on the limbs, elevating the limb can also reduce blood loss.

If undertaking a procedure in a suitable territory (non-end arteries), use of local anaesthetic with adrenaline may reduce bleeding, e.g. removing a sebaceous cyst from the scalp. Remember, injection of adrenaline is contraindicated in an end arterial territory such as the hallux. The use of tourniquets is beyond the scope of this book, except in the context of an ingrown toenail. It is important to keep total tourniquet time to a minimum.

## Diathermy for haemostasis

Electrocautery can be used to achieve haemostasis (Figure 23.1b). This generally consists of the operating surgeon holding the bleeder in a toothed forceps and asking the assistant to 'buzz' – the assistant touches the diathermy tip to the end of the forceps with the blue button and the vessel is coagulated.

## Ligation or suture ligation

The principle of ligation for haemostasis dates back as far as ancient times. There are situations where ligation (Figure 23.2) or suture ligation (Figure 23.3) is more appropriate than electrocautery:

- When diathermy fails to control the bleeding
- When the bleeder is close to an important structure that must not be diathermied
- For large or significant vessels.

In general, suture ligation is used for large or significant vessels or if simple ligation has failed, and simple ligation is used as the primary method for smaller vessels.

### Ligation

1 To ligate a vessel, grasp the vessel in an artery or mosquito forceps.

2 Use a braided absorbable ligature (3-0 for minor surgery) and ensure it is fully around the vessel before tying.

3 Avoid avulsing the vessel by being gentle and avoiding excessive shearing movements.

4 Tie the ligature around the vessel and use your index or middle finger to guide the knot down onto the vessel.

5 Ask your assistant to remove the artery clip as you tighten the first knot.

6 Place at least three square knots when tying a vessel.

### Suture ligation

1 To suture ligate a vessel, grasp the vessel in an artery or mosquito forceps.

2 Use a braided absorbable suture (3-0 for minor surgery).

3 Make a figure of eight around the vessel and then tie the suture.

4 Avoid avulsing the vessel by being gentle and avoiding excessive shearing movements.

5 Tie the ligature around the vessel and use your index or middle finger to guide the knot down onto the vessel.

6 Ask your assistant to remove the artery clip as you tighten the first knot.

7 Place at least three square knots when suture ligating a vessel.

## What to do if haemostasis cannot be achieved?

If haemostasis cannot be achieved, ensure to focus on the patient as a whole and apply resuscitation principles instead of fixating only on the wound.

1 Apply pressure.

2 If you have an anaesthetist, inform them what's going on and explain the urgency of the situation

3 Call for help.

- If you don't have an anaesthetist, consider if you need one and call for one if needed early.
- If you cannot achieve haemostasis, call for senior help to achieve haemostasis
- Call for assistants- without a good assistant, it is difficult to deal with problems- good retraction and lighting is essential
- If you are in the community, consider whether transfer to a hospital setting is indicated

4 Blood products: cross match the patient and inform the haematology laboratory if bleeding is profuse

5 Correct coagulopathy, ensure the patient is warm.

6 Optomise lighting and retraction

7 When you can see a bleeder, control it then consider ligation, suture ligation or simply cautery.

8 When you cannot see the bleeder, consider extending your incision to gain good visualisation.

9 If you cannot get control of the bleeding, apply firm pressure until more help arrives.

# 24 Hypertrophic and keloid scarring

**Figure 24.1** Features of hypertrophic versus keloid scars

**Hypertrophic scars**

Usually stay within the confines of the precipitating trauma

Can occur after major wounds (e.g. following surgery, burns, trauma)

Elevated, thickened appearance. Often red, pruritic or painful

Usually develop rapidly after cutaneous trauma

Improve naturally and gradually (may take up to 2–5 years)

Often regress with therapy

Mostly on extensor surfaces of joints or areas of tension

**Keloid scars**

Invade surrounding, clinically normal skin

Can occur after major wounds, and even following trivial injuries (e.g. injections)

May be pruritic and painful

Develop slowly but continue to enlarge for months to years

Do not resolve naturally

Tend to recur during or after treatment

Mostly arise on the sternum, shoulder, earlobe and cheek

*Minor Surgery at a Glance,* First Edition. Edited by Helen Mohan and Desmond Winter. © 2017 John Wiley & Sons, Ltd. Published 2017 by John Wiley & Sons, Ltd.

# What are they?

Hypertrophic and keloid scars are types of abnormal wound healing.

They are medically benign but are both psychologically and socially problematic. Hypertrophic scars and keloids may arise due to any insult to the deep dermis, including lacerations, abrasions, surgeries and burns. Incidence rates vary widely, being as high as 91% following a burn injury.

Clinical definition:
• Hypertrophic scars usually stay within the confines of the original wound
• Keloid scars extend beyond the boundaries of the original scar, and invade normal surrounding tissue. They do not regress spontaneously, and they tend to recur following excision.

## Distinguishing hypertrophic scars from keloids

Keloids occur more frequently in individuals with darker skin, with African-Americans being particularly susceptible. Both males and females are equally affected. Keloids occur most often between the ages of 10 and 30, and are less frequent at the extremes of age. Table 24.1 compares key features of hypertrophic and keloid scars. However, it is important to note that there can be some overlap between both conditions.

All patients undergoing minor surgery should be counselled regarding scar formation and the risk of keloid scar with poor cosmesis. Options for managing keloid scars include intralesional steroid injection (e.g. triamcinolone), topical silicone dressing therapy and revision. If in doubt, ask a plastic surgeon for advice or opinion.

### Further reading

Bock O, Schmid-Ott G, Malewski P, Mrowietz U. Quality of life of patients with keloid and hypertrophic scarring. *Archives of Dermatological Research* 2006; 297: 433–438.

Edriss AS, Mestak J. Management of keloid and hypertrophic scars. *Annals of Burns and Fire Disasters* 2005; 18: 202–210.

Leventhal D, Furr M, Reiter D. Treatment of keloids and hypertrophic scars: a meta-analysis and review of the literature. *Archives of Facial Plastic Surgery: Official Publication for the American Academy of Facial Plastic and Reconstructive Surgery, Inc and the International Federation of Facial Plastic Surgery Societies* 2006; 8: 362–368.

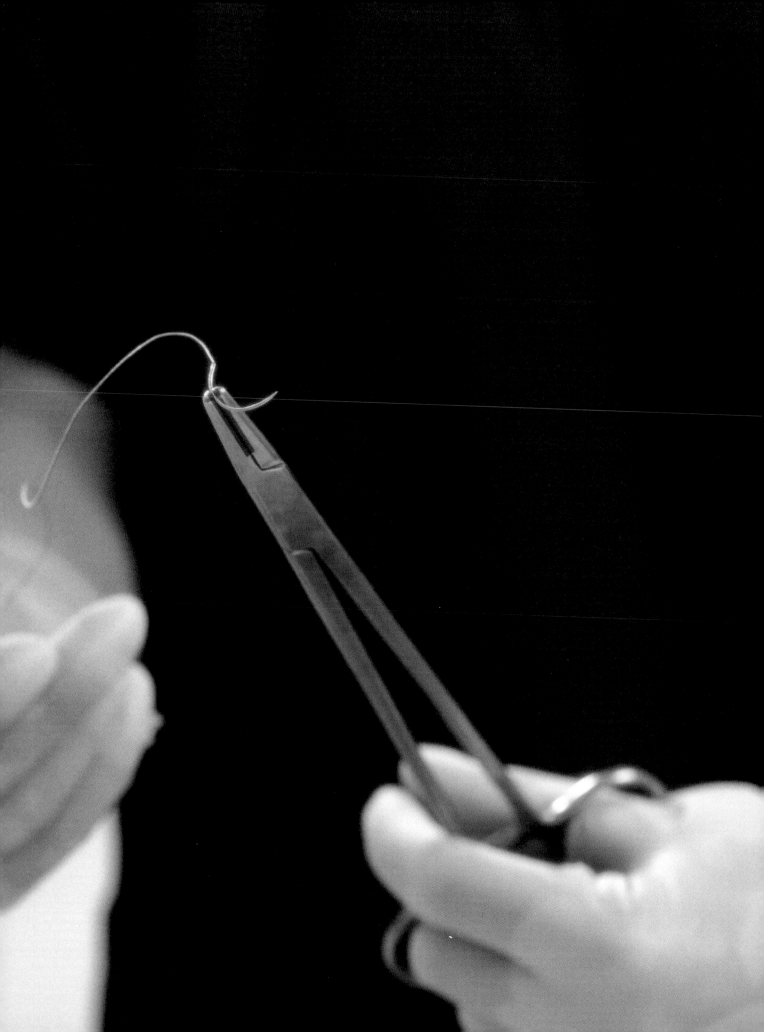

# Practice of minor surgery

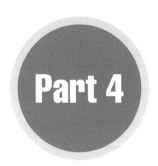

**Part 4**

## Chapters

# 25 Biopsy techniques

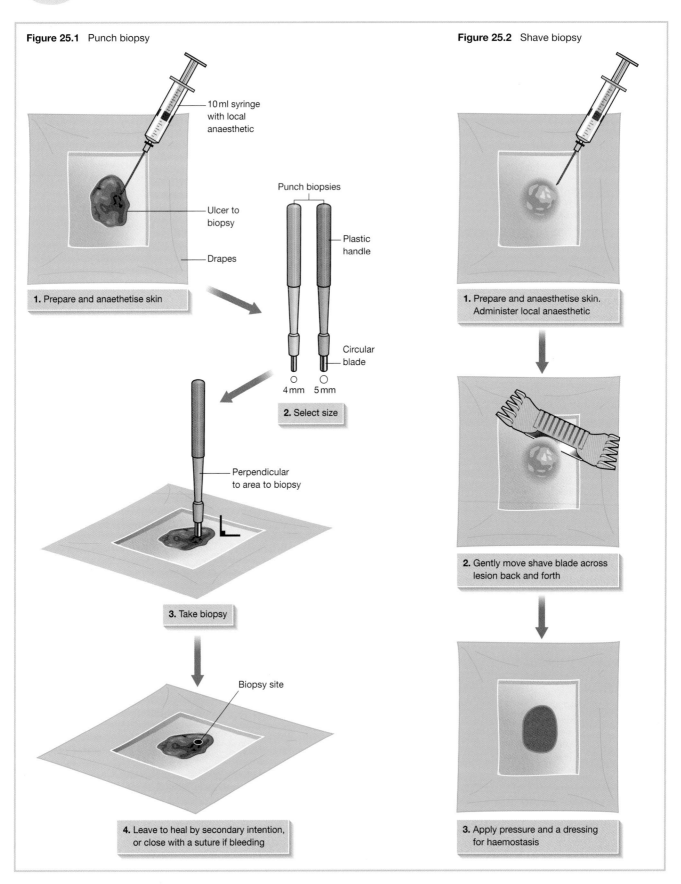

**Figure 25.1** Punch biopsy

10 ml syringe with local anaesthetic

Ulcer to biopsy

Drapes

**1.** Prepare and anaethetise skin

Punch biopsies

Plastic handle

Circular blade

4 mm  5 mm

**2.** Select size

Perpendicular to area to biopsy

**3.** Take biopsy

Biopsy site

**4.** Leave to heal by secondary intention, or close with a suture if bleeding

**Figure 25.2** Shave biopsy

**1.** Prepare and anaesthetise skin. Administer local anaesthetic

**2.** Gently move shave blade across lesion back and forth

**3.** Apply pressure and a dressing for haemostasis

*Minor Surgery at a Glance*, First Edition. Edited by Helen Mohan and Desmond Winter. © 2017 John Wiley & Sons, Ltd. Published 2017 by John Wiley & Sons, Ltd.

# Introduction

The aim of a biopsy is to sample tissue to obtain a diagnosis or guide further management.

**Biopsy:** Obtains a tissue sample for histology with architecture of the tissue preserved.

**Fine needle aspirate:** Aspirates cells for cytology. Fine needle aspiration is beyond the scope of this book.

# Biopsy techniques

## Types of biopsy

Many different types of biopsy exist, depending on the context and what information you are hoping to obtain from the biopsy.

**Excisional biopsy:** This is when the area of interest is removed entirely via a total excision.

**Incisional biopsy:**
1 Punch biopsy – this uses a round or elliptical blade to excise a cylinder of tissue.
2 Shave biopsy – this removes a thin superficial slice of tissue (e.g. in seborrhoeic keratosis).
3 Core biopsy – this uses a hollow needle to obtain a slender core of tissue and is often used in the diagnosis of breast cancer, etc. An in-depth discussion of core biopsy is beyond the scope of this book.
4 Wedge biopsy – this is when a piece of tissue is removed using a scalpel with the aim of taking a large piece of tissue sufficient for diagnosis.

## When to perform an incisional biopsy versus to excise?

**Excisional biopsy:** A lesion with features of cancer should be excised where possible (see Chapter 27).

**Incisional biopsy:** This is useful in a number of settings.
1 For large lesions that would be cosmetically deforming to remove and which will only be removed in the setting of malignancy.
2 To obtain a diagnosis of a skin disorder (e.g. hidradenitis suppurativa).
3 Where repeated biopsy can be a useful therapeutic strategy (shave biopsy).
4 Where the suspicion of malignancy is low but needs to be looked for and excision is not a sensible option (e.g. a chronic leg ulcer).

## Anatomical areas for caution

Be aware of the risk of hitting underlying structures when performing a biopsy. For example, the temporal artery, the facial nerve and the peroneal nerve. The posterior triangle of the neck carries a risk of damaging the accessory nerve if dissecting deeply. (See Chapter 29 on the head and neck for further details.)

## Punch biopsy

Punch biopsy is an easy-to-perform technique that can be carried out in the minor surgery setting or the clinic setting (Figure 25.1). A punch biopsy is usually an incisional biopsy technique. It involves using a circular blade pressed firmly into the tissue to obtain a cylindrical sample. Usually this is used for skin biopsies. An advantage is that it obtains epidermis and underlying dermis with the architecture preserved.

### Punch biopsy technique
1 Use skin preparation for an aseptic technique.
2 Administer local anaesthetic using an orange (25 gauge) or blue (23 gauge) needle.
3 Select the blade size – punch biopsy needles come in a number of different sizes (e.g. 3 mm, 4 mm and 5 mm). The size refers to the circumference of the biopsy. In general, the wider the biopsy the better for diagnostic purposes. However, in cosmetically sensitive areas, a narrower biopsy may be selected.
4 Press the circular blade against the skin area due to be biopsied, holding the skin taught. When selecting the area to be biopsied, for friable lesions select the edge so that you can close it with normal skin.
5 Gently but firmly twist the blade to obtain the biopsy.
6 If the tissue biopsy does not dislodge from the tissue when the circular blade is withdrawn, it may be necessary to hold the tissue with a forceps and use a scalpel to sever remaining connections.
7 In general, close punch biopsies with an appropriate suture (e.g. 5-0 non-absorbable or absorbable suture). Suture to normal skin.
8 Send biopsy to the lab – usually in formalin, and ensure it is appropriately labelled.
9 If the biopsy sample remains in the punch cylinder remove it with a fine forceps or needle.

## Shave biopsy

Shave biopsy consists of taking off a superficial slice of tissue (Figure 25.2). This is suitable for raised lesions. This technique does not sample deeper layers of tissue and is not suitable for suspicious lesions. It is ideal for seborrhoeic keratosis.

### Shave biopsy technique
1 Use skin preparation for an aseptic technique.
2 Administer local anaesthetic.
3 Use a scalpel or a specially designed shave blade to take the superficial layer of skin off the lesion.
4 Send for histology.
5 Apply pressure to achieve haemostasis. Suture closure is not required (usually).

### When 'not' to biopsy

There are several settings when extreme caution should be exercised prior to biopsy.

To achieve clear margins in soft tissue sarcoma, excision of the biopsy tract is necessary. Therefore, if there is any suspicion of soft tissue sarcoma, imaging should be conducted first and biopsy should only be undertaken following liaison with the sarcoma centre/surgeon. If a melanoma is suspected, then excision (not punch) biopsy is indicated unless very large, while lentigo maligna may be sampled with punch biopsy in some circumstances. If in doubt, ask for experienced or specialist advice or assistance.

# 26 Benign and premalignant skin lesions

**Figure 26.1** (a) Seborrheic keratosis
Source: By James Heilman, MD (own work) [GFDL by CC BY-SA 4.0] via Wikimedia Commons

(b) Cornu cutaneum
Source: By Lmbuga (own work) via Wikimedia Commons

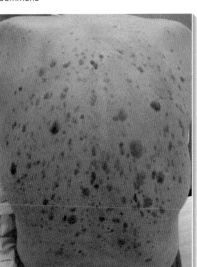

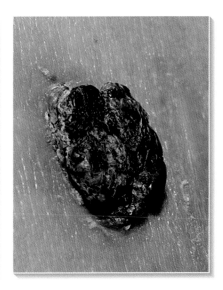

**Figure 26.2** Keratin horn
Source: By Klaus D. Peter, Gummersbach, Germany (own work) [GFDL by CC-BY-3.0-DE] via Wikimedia Commons

**Figure 26.3** Actinic keratosis
Source: By Eray Copcu1, Nazan Sivrioglu1m and Nil Culhaci via Wikimedia Commons

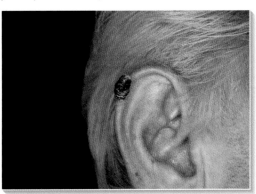

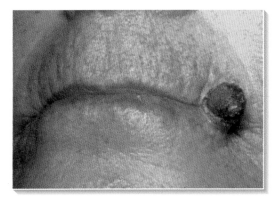

**Figure 26.4** Keratoacanthoma
Source: By Jmarchn (own work) [GFDL by CC-BY-SA-3.0] via Wikimedia Commons

**Figure 26.5** Bowen's disease
Source: By Klaus D. Peter, Gummersbach, Germany (own work) [GFDL by CC-BY-3.0-DE] via Wikimedia Commons

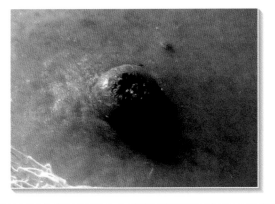

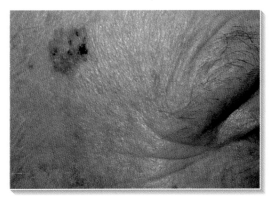

*Minor Surgery at a Glance*, First Edition. Edited by Helen Mohan and Desmond Winter. © 2017 John Wiley & Sons, Ltd. Published 2017 by John Wiley & Sons, Ltd.

## Introduction

This chapter aims to provide a snapshot of commonly encountered skin conditions in the minor surgical setting, rather than an exhaustive overview. Consult dermatology texts for more details. Dermoscopy is useful with appropriate training, but many lesions require biopsy for diagnostic confirmation.

## Benign pigmented lesions

The main indication for removal of a benign pigmented lesion is to exclude a melanoma. There are a number of benign pigmented lesions, including moles and freckles.

### Moles:
- Congenital naevi
- Junctional naevi
- Compound naevi
- Intradermal naevi
- Spitz naevi
- Atypical naevi.

### Freckles:
- Solar lentigo.

If moles or freckles display any suspicious features (see chapter on melanoma), they should be removed with an excisional biopsy where possible.

## Seborrhoeic keratosis

Seborrhoeic keratosis is a benign skin condition characterised by raised, scaly, brownish coloured plaques that are of a waxy consistency (Figure 26.1a). They are not premalignant. The main indications for removal or biopsy is to exclude sinister lesions, for cosmetic purposes, or if catching in clothing causing irritation. Cryosurgery, diathermy excision or formal excision are sometimes used, but shave excision is the ideal method for biopsy and removal (Figure 25.2).

## Pyogenic granuloma

This is a lobular capillary haemangioma. They can bleed easily and become painful. They commonly occur in pregnancy and recede post-partum. In non-pregnant patients, excision-using diathermy is commonly used. Note, it is a misnomer as it is neither pyogenic (producing pus) nor a granuloma.

## Skin tag

A skin tag, or acrochordon, is a benign protrusion of skin that has no malignant potential. The main indication for removal is for cosmetic purposes or if catching on clothes. In general, they are easy to remove by simply decapitating them at the base with either a scalpel or diathermy under local anaesthesia. Closure with a suture may not be required depending on the size of the base.

## Keratin horn

A keratin horn is a cutaneous horn (cornu cutaneum) of keratinised epithelium (Figure 26.2). Although benign, up to 20% of keratin horns have a malignant or premalignant condition, i.e. carcinoma or actinic keratosis (Figure 26.3), at their base. Therefore, treatment strategies should consist of excision of the base rather than just removing the horn. They mainly occur in older patients.

## Keratoacanthoma

This is a rapidly growing skin lesion considered by many to be a variant of squamous cell carcinoma (SCC), although not associated with distant metastases to the same extent (Figure 26.4). It originates in the sebaceous glands beside hair follicles. There is rapid growth over a number of months followed by spontaneous resolution in many cases. Keratoacanthomas most commonly occur in sun-exposed areas. Shave biopsy is not appropriate as it is difficult to differentiate it from SCC. Therefore, excisional or punch biopsy is a better option. The mainstay of treatment is excision. Moh's micrographic surgery, radiotherapy or topical therapies are treatment strategies for invasive skin tumours that are beyond the focus of this book.

## Actinic keratosis

This is a premalignant skin condition (Figure 26.3) which can progress to SCC. It is more common in patients on immunosuppressants. It has a scaly appearance and occurs in sun-exposed areas. Diagnosis is clinical and may require biopsy for confirmation. Treatment is generally with topical 5-fluorouracil therapy with surveillance to out rule development of SCC. Other treatments described include topical NSAIDS, cryotherapy, photodynamic therapy, laser and diathermy.

## Bowen's disease

This condition is SCC *in situ*, with no disruption of the dermal–epidermal junction (Figure 26.5). It is associated with sun-exposure, radiotherapy and Human Papillomavirus (HPV). Common sites for Bowen's are the face, head and neck, legs and genitalia. It usually occurs in older patients. Bowen's disease often appears as a scaly patch, and can mimic other benign skin lesions. Progression to SCC is more common in Bowen's disease of the penis or vulva, occurring in 10% compared to 3–5% of Bowen's disease arising elsewhere. Punch biopsy may be performed to establish the diagnosis if there is diagnostic uncertainty. Options for treatment include excision, photodynamic therapy, curettage, cryotherapy, topical 5-fluorouracil or imiquimod. See dermatology guidelines for further details.

## Dermatoses

Skin conditions such as psoriasis, eczema and so on may require punch or shave biopsy to confirm a diagnosis. Always consider dermatoses in the differential for a skin lesion and consider dermatology referral where appropriate. Always consider premalignant lesions in dermatoses that fail to respond to steroids and consider biopsy. In-depth discussion of dermatoses is beyond the scope of this book.

### Further reading

Morton CA, Birnie AJ, Eedy DJ. British Association of Dermatologists' guidelines for the management of squamous cell carcinoma *in situ* (Bowen's disease). *British Journal of Dermatology* 2014; 170(2): 245–260.

# 27 Melanoma

**Figure 27.1** Margin of excision for excisional biopsy

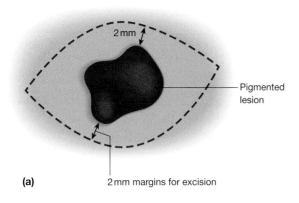

(a)

2 mm

Pigmented lesion

2 mm margins for excision

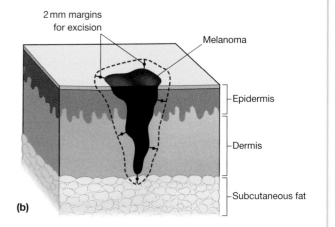

(b)

2 mm margins for excision

Melanoma

Epidermis

Dermis

Subcutaneous fat

**Figure 27.2** Orientation suture

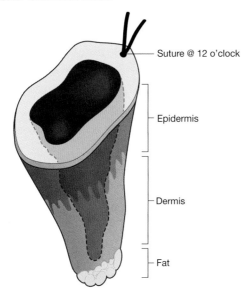

Suture @ 12 o'clock

Epidermis

Dermis

Fat

**Figure 27.3** Breslow thickness

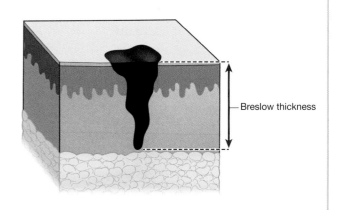

Breslow thickness

*Minor Surgery at a Glance*, First Edition. Edited by Helen Mohan and Desmond Winter. © 2017 John Wiley & Sons, Ltd. Published 2017 by John Wiley & Sons, Ltd.

**P**igmented lesions pose a particular diagnostic difficulty. Whilst the majority are benign naevi (naevus = an increased number of melanocytes concentrated in an area of skin causing pigmentation) they must be differentiated from malignant melanoma. As clinicians we have to decide whether a pigmented lesion requires excision or not and the following features should raise suspicion of a malignant melanoma:

**A. A**symmetry
**B.** Irregular **Bo**rder
**C.** Change in **C**olour / heterogeneity of colour
**D.** Increasing **D**iameter
**E. E**levation / ulceration / bleeding.

If a suspicious lesion is identified a full skin examination should be performed with documentation of the site and size of other pigmented lesions.

## Malignant melanoma

Malignant melanoma is a skin cancer caused by malignant transformation of melanocytes. It is the most fatal form of skin cancer. There are different forms of cutaneous malignant melanoma:

1 Superficial spreading
2 Nodular
3 Amelanotic
4 Acral lentiginous
5 Lentigo maligna.

## Excisional biopsy and margins

A full thickness skin biopsy to include all of the tumour with a 2 mm margin of normal skin on all sides and a cuff of subdermal fat should be performed for clinically suspicious pigmented lesions. This allows pathological tumour staging. Incisional/punch biopsies are only acceptable for lentigo maligna affecting the face or acral melanoma. For subungal melanoma the nail should first be fully removed before biopsy is performed. It is not recommended to prophylactically excise pigmented lesions without suspicious features.

## Procedure of excisional biopsy

1 Mark area to be excised preoperatively with at least a 2 mm margin (Figure 27.1a).
2 Aseptic technique as previously described should be used when performing all excisional biopsies.
3 Local anaesthetic should be infiltrated into the intradermal plane as previously described.
4 Incise along marked outline through ellipse of skin with scalpel blade at 90 degrees to skin at all times to prevent bevelling of scalpel and ensure a full 2 mm perimeter of clear margin throughout all planes of excision (Figure 27.1b).
5 Place a stay suture in the excised specimen to orientate the axis of excision to guide wider excision of margins if required before placing the specimen into formalin (Figure 27.2).

6 Closure of skin should be performed as standard with closure technique and suture material chosen based on size of defect and anatomical location.

## Wider excision of margins

Table 27.1 shows the recommended margins of excision for malignant melanoma base on Breslow thickness (Breslow thickness = measurement in millimeters of the distance between the upper layer of the epidermis and the deepest point of tumour penetration, see Figure 27.3).

**Table 27.1** Recommended margins of excision

| Breslow thickness | Full excision margin |
| --- | --- |
| *in situ* | 5 mm |
| <1 mm | 1 cm |
| 1.01–2.01 mm | 1–2 cm |
| 2.1–4.0 mm | 2–3 cm |
| >4 mm | 3 cm |

## Referral to specialist skin cancer multidisciplinary team

As a general rule all melanoma patients should be referred to a specialist skin cancer multidisciplinary team for consideration of further management. This is particularly important in the following situations:

1 All patients requiring a sentinel lymph node biopsy (Breslow thickness ≥1 mm).
2 Patients with multiple or recurrent melanoma or metastatic melanoma or skin lesions of uncertain malignant potential.
3 Any patient who may be eligible for available clinical trials.
4 Patients with giant congenital naevi with suspicion of malignant transformation.

## Staging

Sentinel lymph node biopsy is the most important staging investigation in patients with melanoma of ≥1 mm. There is no evidence for further imaging if the sentinel node is negative. If positive a CT thorax, abdomen and pelvis with or without CT brain is indicated to rule out further distant metastases. Further investigations should be decided upon by a specialist skin cancer multidisciplinary team (PETCT/MRI/isotope bone scan).

### Further reading

Marsden JR, Newton-Bishop JA, Burrows L, et al. Revised UK guidelines for the management of cutaneous melanoma 2010. *British Journal of Dermatology* 2010: 163; 38–256.

# 28 Non-melanoma skin cancers

**Figure 28.1** Basal cell carcinoma (BCC)

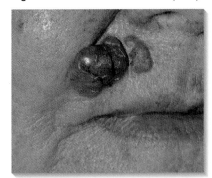

**(a)** Nodular BCC

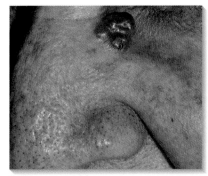

**(b)** Pigmented BCC

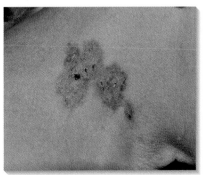

**(c)** Superficial BCC

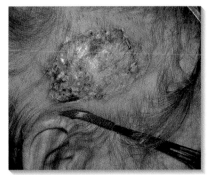

**(d)** Morophoeic BCC

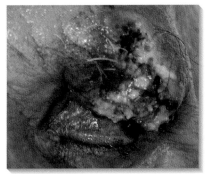

**(e)** Advanced BCC

**Figure 28.2** Squamous cell carcinoma (SCC)

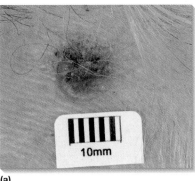

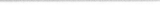

**(a)**

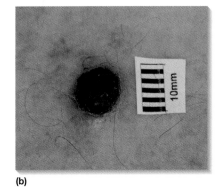

**(b)**

Source: Griffiths, C, et al., eds. *Rook's Textbook of Dermatology, 4 Volume Set*. John Wiley & Sons, 2016.
Reproduced with permission of John Wiley & Sons Ltd.

*Minor Surgery at a Glance*, First Edition. Edited by Helen Mohan and Desmond Winter. © 2017 John Wiley & Sons, Ltd. Published 2017 by John Wiley & Sons, Ltd.

# Introduction

Skin cancers can be divided into melanoma and non-melanomas. Cutaneous cancers are the most common human neoplasms with non-melanoma skin tumours (NMSC) accounting for majority of these. Melanomas are discussed in Chapter 27.

NMSC includes basal cell carcinoma (BCC) (Figure 28.1) and squamous cell carcinoma (SCC) (Figure 28.2), with the former being the most prevalent of all cutaneous cancers.

The incidence of NMSC is rising and identification of these lesions is important for timely management.

# Basal cell carcinoma

BCCs are locally invasive malignant epidermal tumours commonly seen in fair-skinned individuals.

The most significant aetiology is genetic predisposition and exposure to ultraviolet radiation. The majority of BCCs are found in the head and neck region but can also be seen in other sun-exposed areas such as the trunk and lower leg. Typical features of a BCC include:

- Raised pearly white or pink lesion
- Rolled edges
- Telangiectasia of surrounding skin.

They are slow-growing tumours and metastasis is extremely rare. However, local tissue invasion can occur through perivascular or perineural routes. These appear as rodent or ulcerated lesions.

# Squamous cell carcinoma

SCCs are the second most common skin cancer. SCCs commonly appear as hyperkeratosis or an ulcerated lesion. They are most commonly found in sun-exposed areas. However, the variance of SCC is not limited to ultraviolet radiation exposure alone and can be seen in the following:

- Radiation
- Immunocompromised
- Transplant patients
- Bowen's disease
- Marjolin ulcer
- Keratoacanthoma-like SCC.

Unlike BCCs, SCC can metastasise to lymph nodes and internal organs.

## Diagnosis of NMSC

A high index of suspicion and clinical experience is required for prompt diagnosis. Any suspicious lesion where a definite diagnosis cannot be made by inspection alone should be biopsied.

It is important to recognise and distinguish NMSC into low- and high-risk lesions. As per NICE guidelines, high-risk NMSC should be referred to specialty centres while low-risk NMSC that can be managed in the primary setting. Associated factors for high-risk BCCs and SCCs (as per NICE guidelines) are specified here:

### High-risk BCC
- Tumour size >2 cm
- Primary closure is not possible

- Micronodular, morepheaform and infiltrative subtypes (histological)
- Immunocompromised patients
- Location at important anatomical locations
- Recurrent or incompletely excised BCC.

### High-risk SCC
- Tumour size >2 cm
- Tumour site – non-sun exposed areas (e.g. perineum or sole of foot) or chronic inflammation.
- Histological depth – >4 mm
- Acantholytic, spindle, desmoplastic subtypes (histological)
- Recurrent.

## Treatment of NMSC

The definitive treatment of NMSC is excision with clear margins. The size of the tumour will dictate how large the excision margin is. The recommended excision margin is 4 mm from the outer border of the lesion. This is extended to above 6 mm, if lesion size is above 2 cm, particularly if this is a biopsy proven SCC. Excised large lesions should be marked with sutures at either 12 or 6 o'clock and 3 or 9 o'clock to help orientate specimen in pathology.

The marked margin can be extended to an elliptical excision if the surgical wound is to be closed primarily. In closure of a wound with a skin graft, the wound can be excised with a clear margin and the defect mapped to a donor site to obtain adequate coverage. Skin grafts can either be split thickness grafts or full thickness grafts depending on the site. The decision for closure of the wound with a skin graft needs to be made preoperatively to allow for correct positioning, anaesthesia and draping of the donor site.

Other treatment options include non-surgical methods such as curettage, cryosurgery and topical medications such as imiquimod 5% and 5-fluorouracil. These treatments require regular follow-up on an outpatient basis to ensure resolution of the lesion. Failure with conservative management will require surgical management as described earlier.

Another surgical method is the Mohs micrographic surgery, which can achieve high cure rates and long-term benefits in recurrent and multiple NMSCs. This involves removing one layer of tissue at a time and examining for tumor cells microscopically during the procedure.

### Further reading

NICE 2010. Improving Outcomes for People with Skin Tumours including melanoma (update). https://www.nice.org.uk/guidance/csg8/resources/improving-outcomes-for-people-with-skin-tumours-including-melanoma-2010-partial-update-773380189 (accessed 20 June 2016).

Motley RJ, Preston PW, Lawrence CM. Multi-professional guidelines for the management of the patient with primary cutaneous squamous cell carcinoma 2009. Update of the original guideline which appeared in *British Journal of Dermatology* 2002; 146: 18–25. http://www.bad.org.uk/library-media%5Cdocuments%5CSCC_2009.pdf (accessed 20 June 2016).

# 29 Neck lumps

**Figure 29.1** Surface anatomy of neck

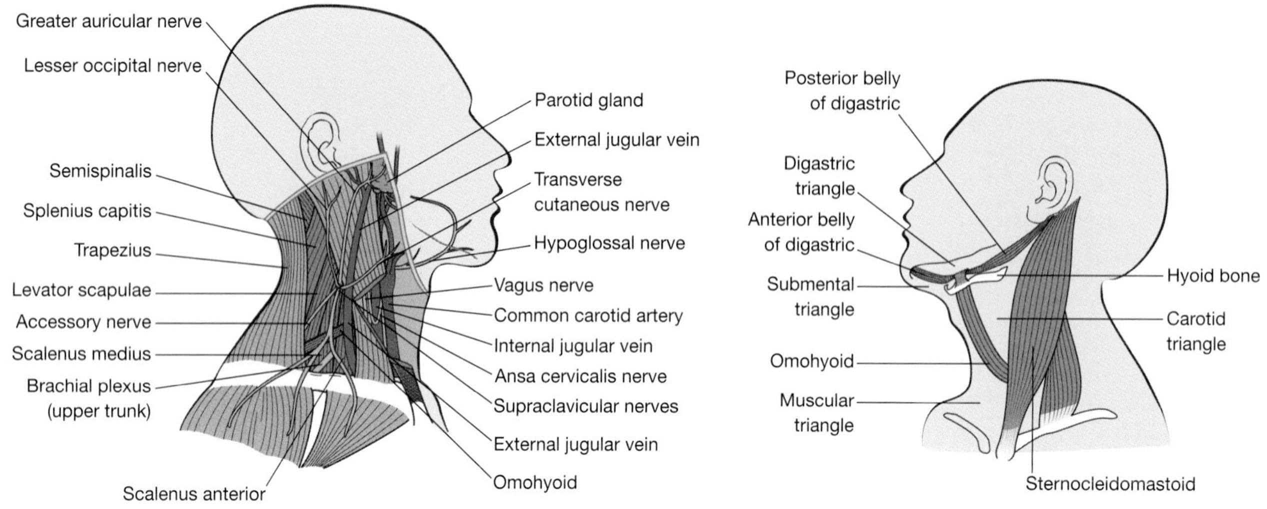

Greater auricular nerve
Lesser occipital nerve
Semispinalis
Splenius capitis
Trapezius
Levator scapulae
Accessory nerve
Scalenus medius
Brachial plexus (upper trunk)
Scalenus anterior

Parotid gland
External jugular vein
Transverse cutaneous nerve
Hypoglossal nerve
Vagus nerve
Common carotid artery
Internal jugular vein
Ansa cervicalis nerve
Supraclavicular nerves
External jugular vein
Omohyoid

**(a)** The main structures in the posterior triangle

Posterior belly of digastric
Digastric triangle
Anterior belly of digastric
Submental triangle
Omohyoid
Muscular triangle

Hyoid bone
Carotid triangle
Sternocleidomastoid

**(b)** Subdivisions of the anterior triangle

**Figure 29.2** Deeper anatomy of neck
Source: Faiz O et al. Anatomy at a Glance, 3rd edn (2011). Reproduced with permission of John Wiley & Sons Ltd.

**(a)** Lateral view

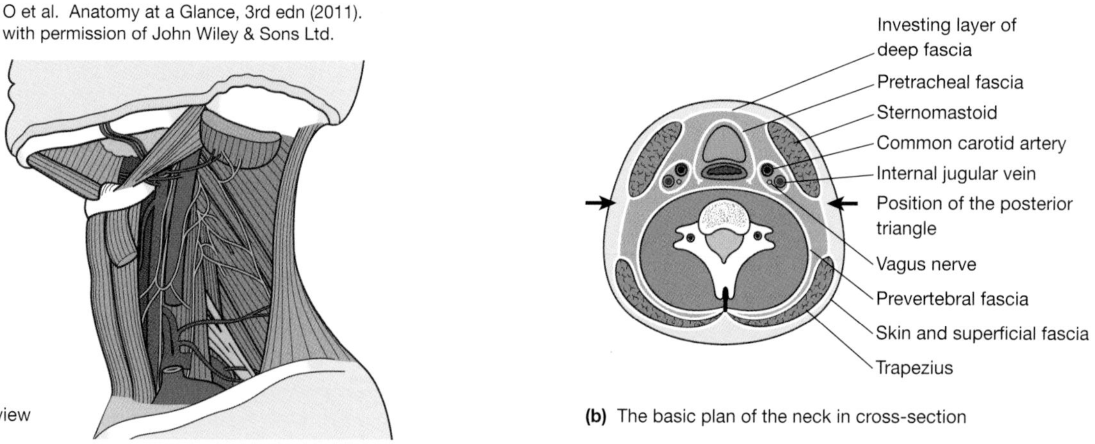

Investing layer of deep fascia
Pretracheal fascia
Sternomastoid
Common carotid artery
Internal jugular vein
Position of the posterior triangle
Vagus nerve
Prevertebral fascia
Skin and superficial fascia
Trapezius

**(b)** The basic plan of the neck in cross-section

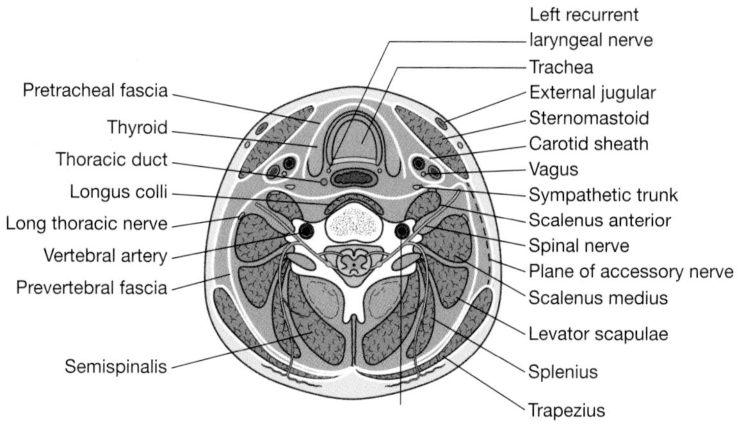

Pretracheal fascia
Thyroid
Thoracic duct
Longus colli
Long thoracic nerve
Vertebral artery
Prevertebral fascia
Semispinalis

Left recurrent laryngeal nerve
Trachea
External jugular
Sternomastoid
Carotid sheath
Vagus
Sympathetic trunk
Scalenus anterior
Spinal nerve
Plane of accessory nerve
Scalenus medius
Levator scapulae
Splenius
Trapezius

**(c)** A more detailed cross-section of the neck

**Figure 29.3** Cervical nodes
Source: Faiz O et al. Anatomy at a Glance, 3rd edn (2011). Reproduced with permission of John Wiley & Sons Ltd.

Buccal
Pre-auricular
Post-auricular
Occipital
Submental
Submandibular
Upper deep cervical
Infrahyoid
Paratracheal
Inferior deep cervical

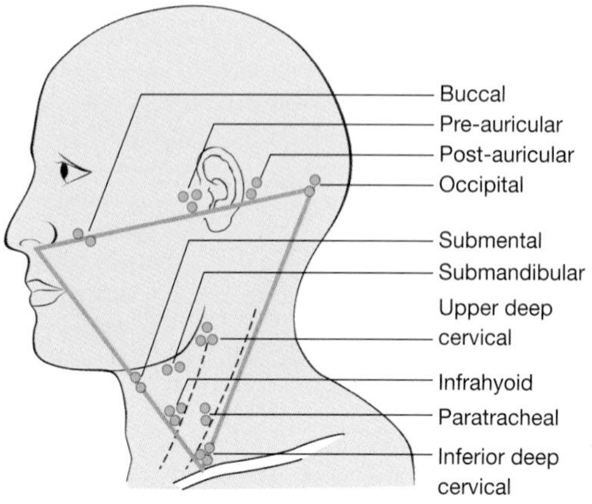

*Minor Surgery at a Glance,* First Edition. Edited by Helen Mohan and Desmond Winter. © 2017 John Wiley & Sons, Ltd. Published 2017 by John Wiley & Sons, Ltd.

# Introduction

Neck lumps are a common clinical finding in all age groups. A careful history and examination can be invaluable in narrowing down a wide range of differential diagnoses. Neck lumps often lie in close proximity to important anatomical structures. For this reason, familiarity with head and neck anatomy is recommended.

# Anatomical considerations

The neck is divided into anterior and posterior 'triangles' (Figure 29.1) by sternocleidomastoid.

Important structures in the anterior triangle include the carotid sheath, thyroid gland and facial nerve branches, while the accessory nerve is at risk with dissection in the posterior triangle (Figure 29.1a and 29.1b). A comprehensive anatomical update is beyond the scope of this book.

# Differential diagnosis

## Midline anterior neck swelling

Thyroid gland pathology (moves with swallowing)

Thyroglossal duct cyst (moves with tongue protrusion)

Dermoid cyst (rare) (midline but does not move with swallowing)

## Anterior triangle neck swelling

Skin/subcutaneous lumps

Lymphadenopathy

Parotid gland pathology

Submandibular gland pathology

Branchial cyst

Cystic hygroma (congential)

Carotid body tumour (rare)

## Posterior triangle neck lumps

Lymph nodes

Skin/subcutaneous tissue lumps

Pharyngeal pouch

# Lymph nodes

Lymphadenopathy is common in a paediatric population, where (or in whom) most are reactive only. Persistence >6 weeks or clinical suspicion should prompt specialist referral.

Reactive lymphadenopathy is also common in adults, but persistence >6 weeks, clinical suspicion, smokers, drinkers or worrying features (dysphonia, dysphagia or persistent sore throat) should prompt referral to a specialist.

# Investigation and management

The history, head and neck examination and features of the lump will determine the appropriate investigations.

Ultrasound scan is the most common first line investigation for neck lumps. It offers the opportunity to perform ultrasound guided fine needle aspiration (FNC) to obtain a cytological profile.

Cross-sectional imaging (CT or MRI) can play a role in helping define neck lumps and their relationship to underlying structures. CT imaging should be extended to include the chest and abdomen where malignancy (e.g. lymphoma) is suspected.

### Further reading

*Head and Neck Cancer: Multidisciplinary Management Guidelines.* 4th Edition. 2011. British Association of Otorhinolaryngology.

# 30 Sebaceous cysts

**Figure 30.1** Incision planning in sebaceous cyst excision

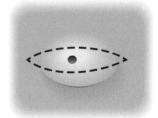

**(a)** Central punctum

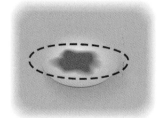

**(b)** Inflamed/scarred

**Figure 30.2** Administration of local for sebaceous cyst

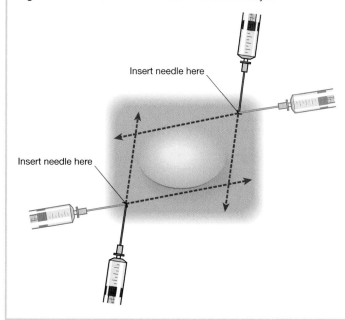

Insert needle here

Insert needle here

## Tips

**1** Avoid excision of an inflamed cyst if possible. These will usually respond to a simple course of antibiotic therapy and can be removed electively at a later date. Note, the cyst may require incision and drainage if an abscess has arisen.

**2** Use local anaesthetic with adrenaline when possible, especially on the scalp to lessen bleeding. Note: local anaesthetic with adrenaline should not be used in extremities/areas supplied by end arteries. Avoid infiltration of the cyst with anaesthetic fluid as this will increase risk of rupture.

**3** Use sharp dissection as much as possible to free the cyst from surrounding skin. Dissect close to the cyst wall for ideal tissue planes.

*Minor Surgery at a Glance,* First Edition. Edited by Helen Mohan and Desmond Winter. © 2017 John Wiley & Sons, Ltd. Published 2017 by John Wiley & Sons, Ltd.

# Introduction

A cyst is an epithelial-lined cavity filled with products of epithelial secretion or products of cell degeneration. Sebaceous cysts, or epidermoid cysts, most commonly affect people in their 20s to 40s and are more common in men (2:1 male:female). These cysts represent a non-cancerous, abnormal proliferation of cells that migrate deep into the skin as a result of implantation of epidermal elements into the dermis following trauma, developmental defect or heredity. The capsule of the cyst is made up of stratified squamous epithelium and contains sebum that has a foul odour when drained.

Sebaceous cysts most commonly present as smooth round bumps commonly found on the scalp, neck, face, chest, and upper back of variable size. They are usually slow-growing, painless, partially moveable lumps beneath the skin. Sebaceous cysts can present acutely with erythema, tenderness and warmth over the affected area of skin.

Indications for removal include:
- A large cyst causing pain or cosmetic issues
- Inflammation/infection-common

# Consent

All surgical procedures come with risk and therefore informed consent must be obtained prior to the procedure. Removal of a sebaceous cyst comes with the general risks associated with removal of all minor skin lesions:
- Bleeding
- Infection
- Haematoma/seroma
- Scar
- While the aim is to completely remove the cyst in its entirety, it must be emphasised that even with precise surgical technique, a sebaceous cyst may recur.

## Skin marking and incision planning

1 Extent and location: Agree site of sebaceous cyst with patient and draw the outline of the circumferential extent of the sebaceous cyst.
2 Skin incision planning: Delineate an ellipse of skin to be removed using a marking pen, ensuring to include any visible punctum in the ellipse. The incision will be determined by the size of the cyst (see Figure 30.1).
3 Positioning: Depending on the location of the cyst (e.g. scalp), shaving a minimal area may be required to get adequate access to the cyst. The patient should be positioned to give adequate, comfortable, easy access to the cyst.

## Local anaesthesia

The skin should be cleaned being careful not to remove site marking. Using 1% lignocaine with adrenaline the local anaesthetic should be infiltrated at four corners of a diamond around the cyst to obtain a field block (see Figure 30.2).

## Equipment required

- Adequate lighting.
- Sterile gloves.
- Skin preparation.
- Sterile drapes, 10 cm × 10 cm gauze pads, suture material, dressing swabs and dressing.
- Standard minor surgery sterile tray containing: scalpel, needle driver, minimum of two curved haemostats, scissors (suture and dissecting), forceps (toothed and non-toothed).

## The procedure

Standard skin preparation should be used.

### Excision

The preferred method involves sharp dissection with the aim of removing the cyst sac and its contents intact without rupture of the cyst and extravasation of its contents. An alternative method involves incising the cyst, expressing the contents and removing the empty sac. The former method is preferred for clean, safe and less malodorous surgery.

### Incision

Using an 11-blade scalpel incise the marked skin in an ellipse. Avoid incising directly over the marking as this may cause tattooing of the skin. Retract the skin edges gently and dissect out the cyst.

### Enucleation

This can be achieved completely with dissection or (if the cyst is small) gentle downward pressure on opposing sides of the skin incision will deliver the cyst once it has been freed from surrounding structures. Ensure that all of the capsule has been removed.

### Skin closure

For small to medium-sized cysts, (up to 2 cm), close with interrupted non-absorbable sutures or with a subcuticular absorbable closure.

For larger cysts, place 3-0 or 4-0 absorbable sutures to take tension off the skin before skin closure.

### Post-operative instruction

**Wound dressing:** Simple dressing (or spray for scalp).
**Specimen:** Although most cysts are benign, the specimen should be sent for histology.
**Follow-up advice:** Simple over-the-counter analgesia usually suffices.

# 31 Lipoma

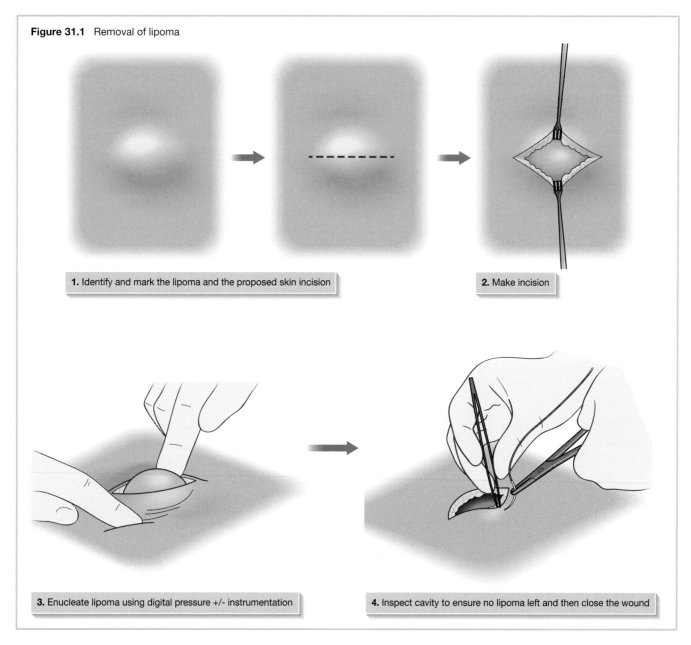

**Figure 31.1** Removal of lipoma

**1.** Identify and mark the lipoma and the proposed skin incision

**2.** Make incision

**3.** Enucleate lipoma using digital pressure +/- instrumentation

**4.** Inspect cavity to ensure no lipoma left and then close the wound

## Preoperative planning
### Considerations: size and site

1 Evaluate the anatomical location:
   - Associated neurovascular structures
2 Assess the structure of the lipoma:
   - Unilobular
   - Multilobular
3 Establish the depth of the lipoma:
   - Subcutaneous
   - Subfascial
   - Intramuscular
4 Determine appropriate anaesthesia:
   - Local anaesthesia (LA) – most lipomata
   - General anaesthesia – large lipomata

5 Determine degree of assistance required:
   - Scrub nurse
   - Surgical assistant

## Informed consent

Discuss the risks, expectations and alternatives of the procedure and in particular highlight:
- Bleeding
- Infection
- Scarring
- Haematoma/seroma
- Neurovascular injury
- Incomplete excision
- Recurrence.

*Minor Surgery at a Glance*, First Edition. Edited by Helen Mohan and Desmond Winter. © 2017 John Wiley & Sons, Ltd. Published 2017 by John Wiley & Sons, Ltd.

## Skin incision

**1 Extent and location**: Draw an outline of the lipoma – this is to agree the site of the lipoma with the patient and to mark the circumferential extent of the lipoma.

**2 Skin incision planning:** Draw the site of the proposed incision prior to LA. Usually, a single straight incision is sufficient, generally about half the length of the lipoma.

## Positioning

- Ensure the patient is comfortable and can maintain the position for the duration of the procedure.
- Ensure you are comfortable and have easy access to the operating field.
- Lighting.

## Equipment

Set up a standard sterile tray, including:
- Forceps (toothed and non-toothed)
- Needle holder
- Dissecting and straight Mayo scissors
- Skin preparation
- 10 × 10 cm gauze swabs
- Diathermy
- Sutures (for example, ethilon to close skin, vicryl for fat sutures and PDS or maxon to close fascia).

## Timeout

Perform timeout according to standard procedures, highlighting concerns and confirming the location of the lipoma to be excised.

## Local anaesthetic

- Usually a field block.
- Use alcohol swabs to clean the wound.
- Begin at the apex of the wound.

### Preparation and draping
- Scrub and apply sterile gloves.
- Clean skin with skin preparation.

# Operative

## Lipoma resection (Figure 31.1)

- Incision: Using the 10- or 11-blade scalpel make a skin incision at the marked site. Avoid incising directly over the mark as it may tattoo the skin.
- Retraction: Ask an assistant to gently retract the skin edges using cats paws/skin hooks, or Langenbeck retractors or by inserting a self-retaining retractor in order to have adequate access to the operative field.
- Dissection: Identify the lipoma and develop a plane by freeing fibrous septae tethering the lipoma by sharp dissection (or diathermy). For multilobular lipomata, each lobule of the lipoma may need to be dissected.

- Enucleation: This is done by gentle downwards pressure on opposing sides of the skin incision using a swab until the lipoma is delivered through the wound. Subfascial or intramuscular lipomas require a more extensive dissection involving incision of the facial sheaths. Free remaining fibrous attachments and remove the lipoma.

## Wound closure

- Ensure adequate haemostasis prior to closure.
- Small lipomata: Close skin using interrupted non-absorbable sutures (e.g. ethilon) or absorbable subcuticular sutures.
- Larger lipomata: Close fascia and subcutaneous adipose layer with absorbable sutures, then close skin as above.

# Post-operative

## Wound dressing

- Simple dressing.

## Specimen handling

- Label specimen including site clearly.
- Send the specimen in formalin for histology.

## Discharge and follow-up advice

- Analgesia as needed.
- Advise on timing and location of suture removal.
- Follow up according to local policy (dressing clinic, GP etc.)
- Advise the patient to return if there are problems and ensure a plan is in place for follow-up of histology results.
- Remove sutures in 10 days for lesions on the back, and 7 days for lesions elsewhere.

# Difficult scenarios

## Inability to enucleate lipoma

- Improve exposure – reposition your assistant/retractors.
- Dissect on or close to the lipoma.
- Lengthen the incision and consider asking for experienced advice/assistance.
- Consider is it a liposarcoma?

## Difficulty with wound closure

- Consider a vertical mattress suture.
- If the wound is under tension, consider elongating the incision. If the incision is elliptical, try and elongate the incision to a smoother ellipse to facilitate closure.
- Consider undermining the edges of the incision to free the skin edge, but avoid devascularising the overlying skin.
   If in difficulty, call for experienced advice/assistance.

# 32 The reconstructive ladder

**Figure 32.1** The reconstructive ladder

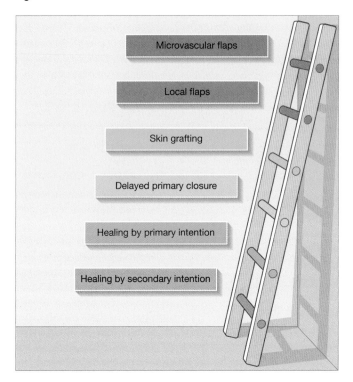

**Table 32.1** Skin grafting

|  | Split-thickness skin graft (STSG) | Full-thickness skin graft (FTSG) |
|---|---|---|
| **Composition** | Epidermis and variable proportion of dermis | Entire epidermis and dermis |
| **Typical donor sites** | Thigh, buttocks | Supraclavicular fossa, post-auricular, abdomen, posterior arm |
| **Potential recipient sites** | Large wounds, burns | On the face and hands |
| **Benefits** | Can cover a large area (e.g. large lower limb defects), contracts in size over time | Better cosmetic outcome, useful around joints as less contraction |
| **Disadvantages** | Produces a significant scar | Size of reconstruction limited by donor site |

*Minor Surgery at a Glance*, First Edition. Edited by Helen Mohan and Desmond Winter. © 2017 John Wiley & Sons, Ltd. Published 2017 by John Wiley & Sons, Ltd.

# The reconstructive ladder

The reconstructive ladder offers a step-wise approach to determine suitable options for wound closure. On the bottom rung of the ladder is the simplest method of healing, progressing to the highest and most complex techniques for closure, microvascular free flap reconstruction (Figure 32.1).

## Healing by secondary intention

Following debridement and cleansing, the wound is left 'open', with dressings applied regularly. This method is the easiest method of wound healing and occupies the lowest rung on the ladder. It tends to result in more obvious scarring. Wounds that are suitable for healing by secondary intention are usually small wounds or wounds which are highly contaminated.

## Healing by primary intention

This is when sutures are used to bring the skin edges together and close the skin defect. These wounds heal much quicker than if they were to heal by secondary intention, and the resulting scar is usually superior.

## Delayed primary closure

This option is considered in wounds that require closure by secondary intention, but in which primary closure is preferred.

Initially, the wounds are treated with dressings, and then an attempt is made to suture the wound at approximately 5 days. It is important that there are no signs of infection when considering delayed primary closure, and that the wound edges can be brought together without tension.

## Skin grafting (Table 32.1)

### Split-thickness skin graft (STSG)

- STSG harvest is usually from the upper thigh. It is carried out using a dermatome, usually set at 8–10/1000 of an inch.
- The dermatome power is turned on before it comes in contact with the patient's skin. It is held at a 45-degree angle to the skin, and pressed firmly against the skin to ensure the graft is harvested evenly. The dermatome is lifted off the skin with the power still on.
- The donor site is dressed.
- The graft is prepared, usually by meshing. Meshing ratios vary from 1.5 : 1 up to 9 : 1 depending on the wound size.
- The recipient site must have a clean, healthy, well-vascularised base. Sites not suitable for STSG include bone without periosteum, tendon denuded of paratenon, vascular or nerve repairs, open fractures, digits or injuries requiring early mobilisation.
- The STSG is inset with the dermis side (shiny side) facing down. It is secured in place, usually with absorbable sutures.
- Immobilisation of the graft is essential to reduce the shear forces that are associated with graft failure.
- The graft is usually left covered until first inspected a few days later.

#### Reasons for STSG graft failure

- Infection (especially beta-haemolytic streptococci).
- Haematoma/seroma.
- Mechanical shearing.
- Co-morbidities (smoking, vascular disease, diabetes).

### Full-thickness skin graft (FTSG)

FTSGs are typically used to close facial or hand wounds.
- It is preferable to use a donor site graft to match the recipient site (e.g. post-auricular graft for reconstruction of an excisional wound on the nose).
- FTSG are marked out using a template of the defect. A scalpel is used to harvest the FTSG, so that the entire dermis and epidermis are included in the graft.
- The graft is then inset at the recipient site using fine absorbable or non-absorbable sutures. A tie-over bolster dressing is typically used to minimise mechanical shear.
- The graft remains dressed until the first inspection a few days later.

# Flap reconstruction

Flap reconstruction is considered when the wound is not suitable for closure by primary or secondary intention (e.g. excessive wound tension), and when skin grafting is not a suitable option (e.g. poorly vascularised bed, exposed bone or tendon at the wound base), and for a better cosmetic outcome. ZY plasty, WY plasty and rotation flaps are examples, but their description is beyond the scope of this book. Similarly, free flaps and microvascular anastomoses are considered not appropriate for a minor surgery text.

#### Further reading

Fernandes R. *Local and regional flaps in head and neck reconstruction: a practical approach*. Oxford, Wiley-Blackwell, 2014.

# 33 Cryotherapy for verrucae (plantar wart)

**Figure 33.1** Liquid nitrogen container

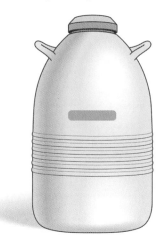

**Figure 33.2** Verruca

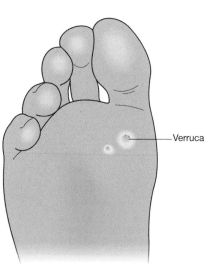

Verruca

**Figure 33.3** Cryotherapy being applied to verruca

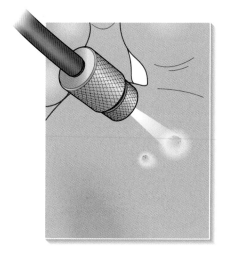

*Minor Surgery at a Glance*, First Edition. Edited by Helen Mohan and Desmond Winter. © 2017 John Wiley & Sons, Ltd. Published 2017 by John Wiley & Sons, Ltd.

# Verrucae

Verrucae (or plantar warts) are a common benign skin condition caused by human papilloma virus (HPV) (Figure 33.1). They are commonly seen in children, most often in 12- to 18-year-olds. The prevalence declines following adolescence and they are very uncommon in infancy. Verrucae are spread via skin-to-skin contact or through contact with contaminated floors (such as in swimming pools and communal changing rooms). Transmission is low but is increased if the epithelial surface is damaged.

Most resolve spontaneously over a period of a few months to years. Factors that affect the rate of resolution include the site and type of verrucae and the age of the patient. Older patients with multiple plantar verrucae have the worst outcome.

Most verrucae are asymptomatic; however, some can become painful, which is one of the most common reasons for seeking treatment. Other indications for treatment include persistent or multiple lesions and unsightly locations (hands, feet and face). Despite the high prevalence of verrucae, the level of evidence on which clinicians can base their treatment is poor.

## Existing treatment options

The purported success of treatments available for verrucae ranges between 30 and 90%. Treatment options include doing nothing, covering the lesion with duct tape, applying topical salicylic acid, cryotherapy, curettage, cautery, and surgical excision. There is no high-level evidence to advocate one treatment above another. The success of treatment is reduced in older patients, long-standing or recurrent verrucae, and in mosaic verrucae (a cluster of verrucae in a small area).

## Cryotherapy

Cryotherapy (sometimes referred to as cryosurgery or cryoablation) takes its prefix from the Greek 'kruos' meaning cold. It is a minimally invasive technique that uses freezing to destroy cells. The mechanism of action is twofold; freezing and thawing directly cause tissue necrosis and then secondary inflammation stimulates the host to mount an immune response.

Cryotherapy should only be used by practitioners who are trained in the technique. The lesion should be first assessed and if there is diagnostic uncertainty, tissue diagnosis should ensue prior to treatment. Although cryotherapy can be used for benign and some malignant skin conditions, its use for malignant skin conditions should only be undertaken by a specialist and is beyond the scope of this book. It should be used with caution in young children, as it can be painful. Cryotherapy should not be used in patients with impaired immunity, diabetes, impaired circulation, collagen disorders, or highly pigmented skin.

### Technique

Liquid nitrogen (Figure 33.2) is the best and most common substance used for cryotherapy due to its low boiling point and ease of use. Other substances, including nitrous oxide and carbon dioxide, were found not to be as effective secondary to their higher boiling points.

There are different delivery devices available including liquid nitrogen spray, dipstick and cold probe. The spray is the most common delivery modality as it is cheap, easy to use, and effective on benign and malignant lesions (Figure 33.3). It is sprayed at a distance of 1 cm for a total duration of 10–30 seconds. The lesion can be palpated after freezing and the cycle repeated to achieve the desired size of effect. Less commonly, a dipstick applicator is used, which involves dipping a cotton-tipped stick into liquid nitrogen and applying it directly to a lesion. This is only suitable for benign skin lesions as the temperatures reached are not low enough for effective treatment of malignant lesions. There is also a probe available which is made from a conductive metal such a copper which can be applied directly to the lesion with a purported higher accuracy; however, this technique is more expensive and time consuming.

## Success of cryotherapy

The varying degrees of success with cryotherapy is thought to be multifactorial. An aggressive technique (meaning longer duration of exposure and repeated cycles) is deemed more effective than gentler regimes. The ideal interval between treatments is not clear; however, side effects are more common with shorter intervals (1–2 weeks), but success of treatment is negatively associated with longer intervals (>4 weeks). The benefit from cryotherapy is thought not to exceed a fourth cycle. Plantar warts are more commonly refractory than warts on other areas of the body, and mosaic verrucae are less likely to completely resolve than simple verrucae. The efficacy of cryotherapy is thought to be enhanced if the keratinised surface of the verruca is scraped off prior to treatment.

Always send samples for histology where there is clinical suspicion of malignancy, topical therapy has failed or there is local progression.

## Side effects of cryotherapy

The most common problem with cryotherapy is pain at the time of the procedure. Some practitioners advocate the use of local anaesthetic tape prior to the procedure, especially for younger children. Blistering and erythema at the treatment site are more commonly seen with repeated cycles and aggressive cryotherapy techniques. Hypopigmentation at the treatment area can occur due to the destruction of heat sensitive melanocytes; however, this is usually temporary. Bleeding and infection at the cryotherapy site is uncommon.

# When to refer to a specialist service

Any skin lesion with an uncertain diagnosis should be referred to secondary care for further assessment. Patients should be referred to a dermatologist when verrucae are resistant to topical treatments and cryotherapy, when cryotherapy is contraindicated, or when they are immunocompromised. Patients with diabetes and verrucae should be referred to a diabetic foot service promptly.

Diathermy excision of verrucae is often considered when repeated episodes of cryotherapy have failed. As this is painful, it is often done under general anaesthesia. Always send the excised specimen for histology as acral (plantar in this case) melanoma may be amelanotic (pigment-free).

# 34 Muscle and nerve biopsy

**Table 34.1** Indications for muscle/nerve biopsy

**(a) Indications or clinical situations for muscle biopsy**

- Suspected myopathy
  - inflammatory (primary or in the context of a systemic autoimmune disease)
  - dystrophy (cause unknown)
  - toxic (cause/extent unknown)
  - metabolic (except hypothyroid myopathy)
  - mitochondrial
  - congenital
  - periodic paralysis
- Refractory myositis
- Malignant hyperthermia
- Suspicion of systemic vasculitis
- Suspected amyloidosis (after negative fat biopsy)
- Parasitic infections

**(b) Indications for nerve biopsy**

- Moderate-severe peripheral polyneuropathy symptoms without a suspected aetiology e.g. diabetes, uraemia and chronic alcohol abuse
- Abnormal electromyography with proven multiple mononeuropathy, or polyneuropathy with reasonable suspicion of:
  - systemic vasculitis
  - amyloidosis (after negative fat biopsy)
  - lymphoproliferative syndromes with poor peripheral blood expression

**Table 34.2** Complications of muscle/nerve biopsy

**Complications (muscle biopsy)**

- Pain
- Bruising/bleeding
- Infection
- Allergy
- Poor healing
- Muscle herniation (rare)
- Keloid scar

**Complications (nerve biopsy)**

- Allergy
- Pain
- Bleeding
- Infection
- Poor healing
- Keloid scar
- Dysthesia/anaesthesia in the region

*Minor Surgery at a Glance*, First Edition. Edited by Helen Mohan and Desmond Winter. © 2017 John Wiley & Sons, Ltd. Published 2017 by John Wiley & Sons, Ltd.

## Introduction

Muscle and nerve biopsies may assist diagnosis in patients with neuromuscular disturbances. A muscle biopsy usually shows a constellation of findings that should be analysed in the context of the patients history, clinical and investigation findings. Nerve biopsies are used mainly to confirm the existence of peripheral nerve involvement in systemic diseases or in non-systemic neuropathy.

## Preoperative considerations

In planning a muscle or nerve biopsy, the surgeon should find out exactly what the relevant specialist is trying to ascertain from the result. It is worth contacting the pathologist pre-operatively to determine how they want the biopsy transported to the lab (e.g. on wet saline soaked gauze). Informed consent must be obtained before commencement.

## Indications and contraindications

Indications for biopsy are summarised in Table 34.1. In the case of suspected systemic vasculitis with peripheral nerve involvement it is recommended to perform a nerve and muscle biopsy to aid diagnosis.

## Open muscle biopsy procedure

1 Based on clinical suspicion, choose a muscle group that is affected by the disease e.g. the deltoid or quadriceps in patients with suspected inflammatory myopathy and ideally choose a symptomatic muscle without atrophy. Avoid muscles with recent trauma (including electromyography needles or intramuscular injections).

2. Mark the proposed incision. The ideal size is 2–4 cm, which can vary depending on the amount of subcutaneous tissue.

3 Apply antiseptic solution. Infiltrate the area with local anaesthetic subcutaneously without reaching muscle tissue. Wait for it to take effect (1-2 minutes).

4 Make the incision with a scalpel (10 blade). Dissect the subcutaneous tissue to the aponeurosis using scissors. Insert a self-retaining retractor to expose the muscle.

5 Clamp with dissecting forceps a small group of muscle fibres to the desired depth (approximately 0.5 cm) then sever the desired length for sampling (approximately 2 cm). Ask your pathologist in advance how much tissue is desired. Take care to avoid excessive handling of the muscle to avoid artefact. Another approach is to use a suture as a sling to select the group of muscle fibers for biopsy, and clamp and divide on either side of the selected length. Take care not to clamp the muscle you intend to use as the biopsy as it will cause artefact. The remaining clamped ends can then be ligated.

6 Ensure adequate haemostasis. Close the muscular fascia with absorbable sutures, then close the skin with interrupted non-absorbable sutures. If subcuticular absorbable skin closure is preferred, then close subcutaneous fat with interrupted absorbable sutures.

## Needle muscle biopsy procedure

Introduced by Bergström in 1962, needle muscle biopsy is suitable for adult and paediatric patients. The advantage over open biopsy is simplicity and speed. In children sedation may be needed and the quadriceps muscle (vastus lateralis) is the preferred site. The skin is prepared in the usual way and both the skin and subcutaneous tissue are infiltrated with local anaesthesia, in the same manner as for open muscle biopsy.

Make a small incision in the skin and insert the Bergström needle with the sliding cannula assembled with the window closed in the muscle. The window is then opened allowing the muscle to go into the window. The needle is then withdrawn and the muscle sample removed. The needle can be reintroduced through the same incision and additional samples can be obtained. After completion of the biopsy, digital pressure is applied. No suture is necessary. Although this procedure is simpler and quicker than open biopsy, nevertheless, the sample is small and orientation in the laboratory can be difficult.

## Nerve biopsy procedure

1 The most common nerves selected for nerve biopsy are cutaneous sensory nerves, e.g. the sural nerve or superficial peroneal nerve in the leg. Specific considerations to discuss with the patient are given in Table 34.2. Having consented the patient, prepare the surgical site as previously described. Choose the most affected nerve and know the precise anatomical location and relations.

2 Mark the site before starting and confirm it with the patient.

3 The ideal incision size is 2–3 cm, which can vary depending on the amount of subcutaneous fat.

4 Locate the nerve (posterior lower leg for sural nerve) wrapped in fat within the neurovascular bundle. To differentiate it from the rest of the neurovasuclar structures, remember it has a pearly colour and flat shape. Often, if the nerve is not too affected, the patient will experience tingling on the region supplied at this stage (foot for sural nerve).

5 Remove 2 cm of nerve, ideally. Do not remove the surrounding adipose or fibrous tissues. It is not necessary to suture the ends. If the manipulation is not painful, there is no need to anaesthetise the nerve for sectioning. However, if nerve manipulation is painful, infiltrate with local anaesthetic.

6 Next, remove a piece of muscle near the nerve, proceeding just as in the previous section. Ensure adequate haemostasis.

7 Close the muscle fascia with absorbable sutures and close the skin as above.

# 35 Ingrown toenail

**Figure 35.1** Schematic of nail anatomy

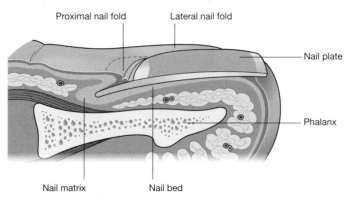

Proximal nail fold — Lateral nail fold — Nail plate — Phalanx — Nail matrix — Nail bed

**Figure 35.2** Application of local anaesthetic

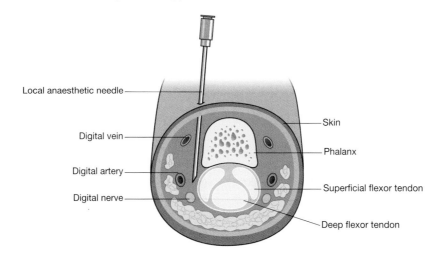

Local anaesthetic needle — Digital vein — Digital artery — Digital nerve — Skin — Phalanx — Superficial flexor tendon — Deep flexor tendon

**Figure 35.3** Ingrown toenail removal

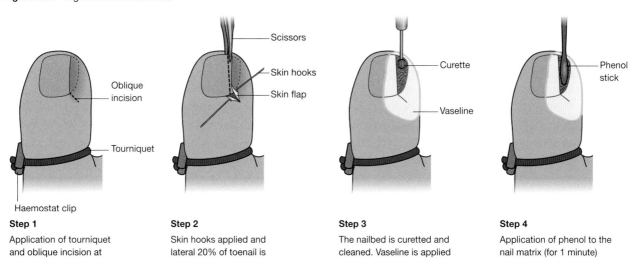

Oblique incision — Tourniquet — Haemostat clip

Scissors — Skin hooks — Skin flap

Curette — Vaseline

Phenol stick

**Step 1**
Application of tourniquet and oblique incision at nail corner

**Step 2**
Skin hooks applied and lateral 20% of toenail is removed

**Step 3**
The nailbed is curetted and cleaned. Vaseline is applied to surrounding tissue prior to phenolisation

**Step 4**
Application of phenol to the nail matrix (for 1 minute)

*Minor Surgery at a Glance,* First Edition. Edited by Helen Mohan and Desmond Winter. © 2017 John Wiley & Sons, Ltd. Published 2017 by John Wiley & Sons, Ltd.

## Introduction and pathogenesis

Ingrown toe nail or onychocryptosis is a frequent minor surgical procedure. It commonly affects the hallux, causing significant discomfort. It occurs typically due to improper trimming resulting in the creation of a barb (spicule) at the lateral nail groove that pierces the periungal epidermis, which penetrates deeper as the nail grows forward. The presence of a foreign body results in an inflammatory reaction with formation of granulation tissue. If persistent can ultimately result in infection and/or abscess formation.

## Aetiology/risk factors

Ingrown toenail is extremely rare in populations that don't wear shoes commonly. The majority of cases are due to improper trimming, but there is also a multifactorial component including poor fitting or narrow pointed shoes; poor foot hygiene or hyperhidrosis; repetitive trauma or excessive running; genetic predisposition or over-curvature of the nail in elderly persons.

## Anatomy

The nail unit comprises the:
- nail matrix
- nail bed
- proximal and lateral nail fold.

The nail matrix contains germinative epithelium from which the nail matrix keratinoctyes differentiate to form the nail plate. The majority of the nail matrix is hidden just proximal to the proximal nail fold. The nail bed which possesses a rich vascular supply extends transversely between both lateral nail folds. It is at the lateral nail fold that is most susceptible to the development of an ingrown toenail. (See Figure 35.1 for schematic illustration of nail anatomy and development of ingrown toenail.)

## Management

### Management options for ingrown toe-nail

Conservative:
- Warm water soaks + proper nail trimming
- Taping
- Packing with cotton wool or dental floss wisps
- Gutter splinting

Surgical:
- Simple nail edge excision
- Partial or total nail avulsion
- Partial nail avulsion/excision with phenol matricectomy (see later and Figure 35.3)
- Partial nail avulsion with sodium hydroxide matricectomy
- Partial matricectomy using electrocautery or carbon dioxide laser ablation
- Surgical excision of nail plate and matrix (Zadik's procedure)

### Conservative management options

**Warm soaks:** Usually for 10-20 minutes. Improves foot hygiene. After soak most apply topical antibiotic ointment (e.g. neomycin, polymyxin B and bacitracin). This is usually repeated until resolution of pain.

**Taping:** Tape is applied to the lateral nail fold resulting in the dermis being retracted away from the offending nail barb (spicule). However this method is cumbersome, with need for repeated application of tape due to slippage of tape because of lack of adhesion to the granulation tissue edge.

**Packing with cotton wool or dental floss wisps:** Wisp is placed under the lateral fold of the ingrown toenail with aid of nail elevator (with or without local anaesthetic). The wisp may be soaked with an antiseptic agent. Over time the nail edge will be displaced from ingrowing, though this may take several months.

**Gutter splint:** A small guard is inserted between the lateral nail margin and the nail fold. Common material used as gutter is an intravenous tube cut lengthwise and placed under local anaesthetic. The tube may be fixed with sutures. Normally it takes 8 weeks for the nail to grow out and inflammation to reside.

### Surgical technique – lateral wedge excision +/– phenolisation

1 Consent: Discuss general risks, benefits and alternatives highlighting the following risks: bleeding, infection, pain, recurrence, abnormal nail appearance/deformity/poor cosmetic result and toe ischaemia (only with prolonged tourniquet use or tight dressing).
2 Timeout: Perform timeout according to standard procedures, highlighting concerns, allergy status and surgical site.
3 Local anaesthetic (LA): Use alcohol swab to clean site. Lidocaine or bupivacanine **without** adrenaline in a digit block fashion (see Figure 35.2). Typically start administration with a 25G needle, then 23G. Approx 7–10 mL of LA is required.
4 Preparation / draping: Position patient with affected foot hanging over edge of bed (supine). Prepare toe with povidone-iodine solution. A tourniquet may be applied – if using a tourniquet, record the time applied and total tourniquet time (Figure 35.3 Step 1).
5 Procedure: Assess adequacy of LA (may need additional anaesthetic). An oblique incision at the proximal corner of nail is made (2–3 mm) – this typically bleeds initially. Skin hooks are applied and the incision deepened down (but not including the nail or nail bed). Identify the lateral 20% of the ingrown nail. Cut the nail and excise the associated nailbed (Figure 35.3 Step 2). The nail bed may be curetted to remove any remaining matrix/granulation tissue off the nail bed from the phalanx.
6. Phenolisation: If using phenol, apply petroleum jelly to the surrounding tissues (Figure 35.3 Step 3). A small pledget of cotton wool soaked in phenol[1] is placed into the nail base defect to destroy any residual matrix (left in place for 1 minute) (Figure 35.3 Step 4). The cotton ball is removed and copious surgical alcohol wash is used to neutralise the phenol. Clean the wound well with gauze and apply microporous dressings to approximate edges. A calcium alginate square is applied and held in place with gauze dressing and roll. Remove the tourniquet if used after some pressure has been exerted by the dressing. Finally check for normal perfusion of the toe.

**Post-operatve care:**
- Oral analgesics
- Elevation post-procedure
- Change bandage 24-hours later – typically in a dressing clinic where the patient is educated on how to clean and apply a bandage. Soaking the bandage in warm water prior to removal minimises discomfort of adhered dried blood.

**Complications:**
- Excessive bleeding – needs compression
- Incomplete matricectomy can result in re-growth of the nail spicule – needs a repeat procedure
- Post-op infection (red, hot swollen toe) – needs oral antibiotics
- Prolonged application of tourniquet can result in distal toe ischaemia – limit tourniquet time to less than 15 minutes
- Nail plate dystrophy – permanent disfiguration (more common with nail plate biopsy).

[1] Phenol is a colourless crystal derived from coal tar. When liquefied, it has both antibacterial and anaesthetic properties. Application of phenol results in denaturation/necrosis of the nail matrix.

# 36 Lymph node excision

**Figure 36.1** An example of inguinal lymphadenopathy

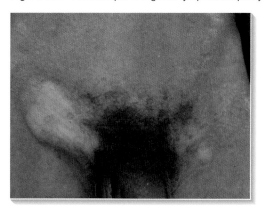

**Figure 36.2** Langer's lines

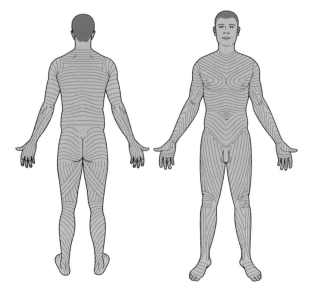

**Figure 36.3** Incision

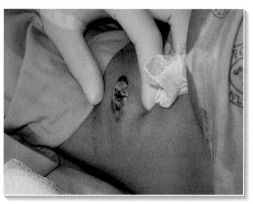

**Figure 36.4** Lymph node appearance

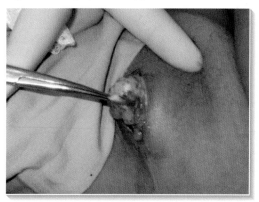

**Figure 36.5** Exposing vascular pedicle

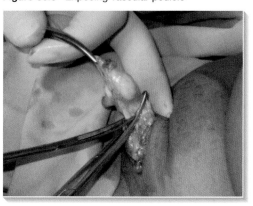

**Figure 36.6** Subcuticular suture

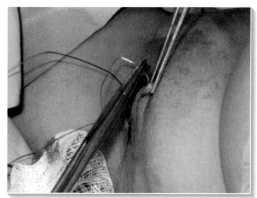

Lymph node excision is a common minor surgical procedure. The primary indication is *diagnostic* – to determine the aetiology of lymphadenopathy, or staging – e.g. inguinal node excision for anal cancer (Figure 36.1) or melanoma. Although the utility of fine needle aspiration has improved, results are often equivocal. Excision of an entire node provides sufficient tissue mass to analyse histological, immunohistochemical and microbiological characteristics and is thus still considered the diagnostic procedure of choice, especially in cases of suspected haematological malignancy.

Abdominal or retroperitoneal lymph node biopsy, and the *therapeutic* and *prognostic* role of lymph node excision in cancer surgery, are beyond the scope of this text.

## Preparation

Although a so-called minor procedure, standard principles of surgical preparation and technique must be respected to avoid the commonest complications. These are haematoma and wound infection, with seroma or lymphocoele, poor scarring and nerve damage also reported.

Although the procedure can usually be carried out under local anaesthetic, this may be problematic for deeper or fixed nodes in awkward locations. General anaesthesia is a perfectly acceptable requirement in these patients, and we prefer it, or a regional block, for axillary dissection.

A clear explanation, sufficient for informed consent, should include discussion with the patient of their operative positioning, particularly regarding neck or shoulder mobility. There may be several lymph nodes, and the surgeon should select one with ease of access and avoidance of dangerous structures. For example, excision in the posterior triangle of the neck is a safer undertaking than in the anterior triangle.

Position the patient comfortably and ensure that adequate lighting is available. For excision in the neck, directing the patient's gaze to the contralateral side will give definition to the sternocleidomastoid muscle. For axillary lymph node excision, having the patient rest the hand of the affected side behind the head will provide ready access to the axilla. The axilla should be shaved.

Prior to full skin preparation, the planned incision site should be infiltrated with adequate local anaesthetic, with adrenaline, after cleaning with alcohol. This allows the anaesthetic to take effect during draping and hand washing. The ampoule can be diluted to ensure adequate volume. Lymph node excision should be a painless procedure.

Instruments should include fine retractors and dissecting forceps and scissors. Electrocautery (mono- or bipolar) should always be available.

## Procedure

The incision should be placed in Langer's lines (Figure 36.2) directly over the lymph node. The length of incision should be sufficient to facilitate an easy dissection (Figure 36.3). A common error is to attempt removal through too small an incision, especially when operating without an assistant. Bleeding and haematoma are the likely consequence, with little aesthetic benefit.

Once through the superficial fat and fascia, the dissection is continued with a fine artery forceps or scissors spreading the tissue transversely and longitudinally, dissecting in the peri-capsular plane of the node. This can be identified by a subtle red hue visible through its translucent capsule (Figure 36.4). The capsule is thin and the node fragile, but by gentle grasping with an atraumatic forceps, the node can be teased free without fracturing the capsule. Traction on the node with an Allis tissue holder, or toothed clamp, is discouraged; rather, patient dissection through an enlarged incision, is preferred. Occasionally, the gland complex may extend into deeper tissues adjacent to major structures making excision of the entire node unsafe. Under these circumstances, partial excision is safer and usually provides sufficient tissue for analysis.

The vascular pedicle, usually located on the underside of the lymph node, should be identified and ligated with an absorbable suture (Figure 36.5). With the lymph node removed, the wound is inspected meticulously for residual bleeding.

The wound can be closed with a single cutaneous suture, or with a deeper soft tissue suture. The cutaneous suture can be continuous or interrupted, with the latter preferred in an area of cutaneous tension or in the axilla with its increased risk of infection (Figure 36.6). An alternative is to approximate the wound edges with an interrupted subcutaneous suture to relieve tension on the subcuticular suture. Apply a simple dressing to complete the procedure.

## Specimen preparation

Discuss with the local pathology service regarding their preferred preparation of excised lymph nodes, which may include sectioning, and placement in separate containers. Generally, samples can be sent fresh for frozen section, fixed in formalin for histological examination and in normal saline for microbiological analysis.

### Further reading

Baigrie RJ, Lymph-node biopsy, in Morris PJ, Malt RA (ed.) *Oxford Textbook of Surgery*. 1st edn. USA: Oxford University Press, 1994; pp 2130–2131.

Blanco JM, Tejero M. Skills in minor surgical procedures for general practitioners, in: OresteCapelli (eds) *Primary Care at a Glance – Hot Topics and New Insights*. Italy: InTech; 2012; pp 101–136.

Giuliano AE, Kelemen PR. Lymph node diagnosis, in: Morris PJ, Wood WC (eds) *Oxford Textbook of Surgery*. 2nd edn. USA: Oxford University Press; 2000; pp 2764–2766.

Hehn ST, Utility of fine-needle aspiration as a diagnostic technique in lymphoma. *Journal of Clinical Oncology* 2004; 22(15): 3046.

# 37 Sclerotherapy

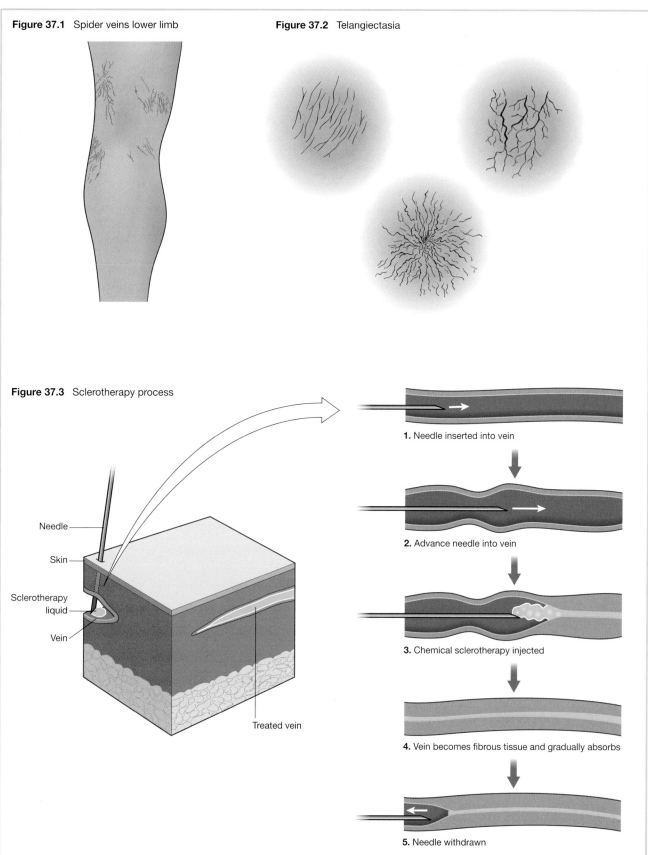

**Figure 37.1** Spider veins lower limb

**Figure 37.2** Telangiectasia

**Figure 37.3** Sclerotherapy process

Needle

Skin

Sclerotherapy liquid

Vein

Treated vein

**1.** Needle inserted into vein

**2.** Advance needle into vein

**3.** Chemical sclerotherapy injected

**4.** Vein becomes fibrous tissue and gradually absorbs

**5.** Needle withdrawn

*Minor Surgery at a Glance*, First Edition. Edited by Helen Mohan and Desmond Winter. © 2017 John Wiley & Sons, Ltd. Published 2017 by John Wiley & Sons, Ltd.

Sclerotherapy is a minimally invasive, percutaneous technique that involves the injection of a chemical irritant into a varicose or spider vein, causing damage and scarring of the vessel with resultant collapse and closure of the vein. The body naturally absorbs the treated vein over a period of weeks. Sclerotherapy has been around in one form or another for well over 100 years and there are descriptions going back much further. This chapter focuses on the use of sclerotherapy for spider/thread veins as the use of sclerotherapy for varicose veins is beyond the scope of this book.

## Indications

Sclerotherapy is commonly used to treat telangiectasias, small spider veins (venous flare) and smaller varicose veins (Figure 37.1 and Figure 37.2), predominantly on the lower limbs. This is most commonly performed for cosmetic purposes. Sclerotherapy can also be used to treat any remnant tributaries after endovenous laser ablation of a saphenous or truncal vessel.

## Considerations

Before offering sclerotherapy to your patient you should clearly document a full medical history including allergies, use of anticoagulants, prior varicose vein interventions and assess risk factors for deep venous thrombosis, such as smoking or use of the oral contraceptive pill.

Check for underlying venous disease on physical exam and any evidence of concurrent thrombophlebitis.

Contraindications include pregnancy, thrombophlebitis, pulmonary emboli, hypercoagulable states, and allergy to the sclerosing agents.

## Consent/risks

Sclerotherapy is a low-risk procedure; however, as it is often performed for cosmetic purposes, it is important that your patient is counselled carefully.

Discuss alternatives to the procedure and emphasise the potential need for repeat procedures. Alternatives include laser treatment for thread veins.

Local adverse reactions to injection sclerotherapy include pain, ulceration, urticaria, hyperpigmentation, and telangiectatic matting at the injection site due to extravasation of the sclerosant or red blood cells. These are mostly transient and resolve within weeks to months.

More serious complications are rare but have been reported and include intense superficial thrombophlebitis and deep venous thrombosis, visual and neurological disturbances (usually in the presence of a patent foramen ovale), cough and anaphylaxis.

New vessels are likely to develop over time and repeat treatment may be necessary in the future. Treatment sessions for the same anatomic locations are carried out at intervals of 4–8 weeks.

## Preparation

### Sclerotherapy agents

The most common agents used are sodium tetradecyl sulfate, polidocanol, glycerin, and hypertonic saline. These all cause endothelial damage by either an osmotic or detergent mechanism. Osmotic agents cause dehydration of endothelial cells through osmosis and detergents are surface-active agents that damage the endothelium by interfering with cell membrane lipids.

## Foam sclerotherapy

Foam sclerotherapy can be used in both larger vessels and in spider veins. It involves mixing a detergent sclerosing agent with a gas (commonly air), resulting in foam formation. The foam preparation is obtained after repeated alternate passages from one syringe to another through a connector. Compared to traditional liquid sclerotherapy, foam sclerotherapy has certain advantages including a smaller volume of the sclerosing agent needed for injection, lack of dilution with blood (dilution decreases efficacy), homogeneous effect along the injected veins, and ultrasound echogenicity.

Specific adverse events are similar to liquid sclerotherapy and include pulmonary symptoms (cough), and visual and neurologic events (in the presence of a patent foramen ovale), localised inflammatory phlebitic reactions and post-treatment hyperpigmentation.

## The procedure

Venous distension is increased in the standing position making identification of spider veins easier, but successful sclerotherapy can be carried out with the patient horizontal (Figure 37.3).
- Ensure excellent lighting.
- Sterilise area with alcohol prep.
- Use 30-gauge needle, insert into vein, bevel up.
- Injection should be precise and slow – each injection should be 0.1–0.4 mL using a 1 mL syringe.

*Severe pain or burning is often a sign of extravasation so stop injecting sclerosant.* In the event of extravasation of sclerosant, some surgeons inject the site with normal sodium chloride solution to dilute the sclerosant.

After the needle is removed, compression with dressings or bandaging is used. The pretibial area and ankle skin have the highest propensity for ulceration. Treatment in these locations should be limited in each session.

## Post-procedure

- Class 1 (20–30 mmHg) compression stockings for 3–4 weeks.
- Low intensity extremity exercises are permitted following the procedure.
- Avoid sun exposure on treated sites for 6 weeks.
- The patient should contact their doctor immediately if they are experiencing increasing pain or if any ulcers are observed at the injection sites.
- Repeat injections, which are frequently needed, are not performed for at least 4 weeks.

Table 37.1 Complications

| Common complications | Uncommon complications |
| --- | --- |
| Bruising | Thrombophlebitis |
| Hyperpigmentation | Tissue necrosis |
| Oedema | Deep venous thrombosis |

# 38 Botulinum toxin

**Figure 38.1** Common sites for botox and filler injection

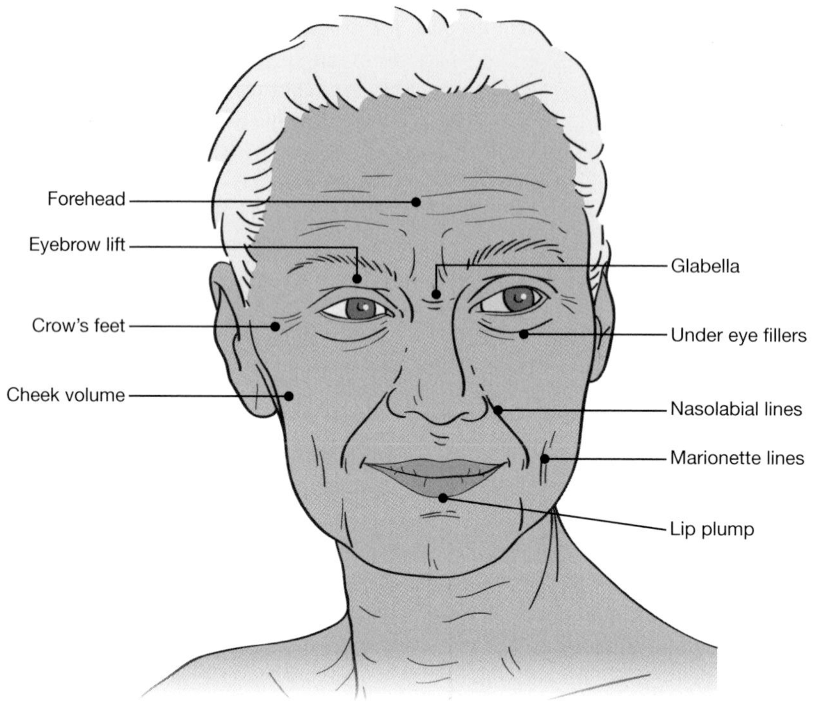

Forehead

Eyebrow lift

Crow's feet

Cheek volume

Glabella

Under eye fillers

Nasolabial lines

Marionette lines

Lip plump

**Figure 38.2** Intradermal injection

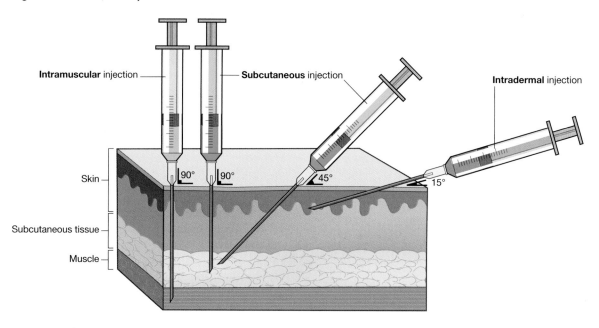

**Intramuscular** injection

**Subcutaneous** injection

**Intradermal** injection

Skin

90° 90° 45° 15°

Subcutaneous tissue

Muscle

*Minor Surgery at a Glance*, First Edition. Edited by Helen Mohan and Desmond Winter. © 2017 John Wiley & Sons, Ltd. Published 2017 by John Wiley & Sons, Ltd.

# Botulinum toxin

Botulinum toxin ('Botox') is an injectable neuromodulator derived from *Clostridium botulinum*. It inhibits neurotransmission at the neuromuscular junction and is used to weaken or paralyse skeletal muscle.

There are multiple medical uses for botulinum toxin. This chapter focuses on cosmetic indications. Other uses include in surgery for an anal fissure, and in the treatment of hyperhidrosis.

Botulinum toxin is widely used in cosmetic surgery (Figure 38.1). Some common indications include:
- Forehead wrinkles
- Glabellar wrinkles (11's)
- 'Crow's feet' wrinkles
- Upper and lower lip wrinkling
- Cobblestone chin
- Excessive gingival show ('gummy smile')

## Dosage

The standard dose for glabellar botox injection is 20 botox units.

## Injection

Microinjection technique – administers low doses superficially, similar to intradermal injections. For forehead wrinkles, typically 100 units of botulinum toxin are resuspended in 2.5 mL of saline. This is drawn up into an insulin syringe and results in 4 units of botox in 100 microlitres of solution. Typically inject 100 microlitres per site 1 cm apart. See Figure 38.2 for sites of injection.

## Side effects

Botox is generally well tolerated but has serious potential side effects. It is therefore of paramount importance that botulinum toxin is only performed by appropriately trained staff in the correct setting. Transient local site effects may occur (swelling and bruising at the injection site). Excessive or improper placement of the toxin can result in functional impairments (e.g. incompetent mouth) or disfigurement, especially a risk of ptosis in the face. Effects are temporary, typically lasting 3 months or less. Intravascular injection of botox can result in paralysis, respiratory arrest and death.

### Further reading

De Maio M, Rzany B (eds). *Botulinum Toxin in Aesthetic Medicine*. Berlin Heidelberg: Springer Verlag, 2007.

Gilchrest BA, Krutmann J (eds). *Skin Aging*. Berlin Heidelberg: Springer Verlag, 2006.

# 39 Tetanus

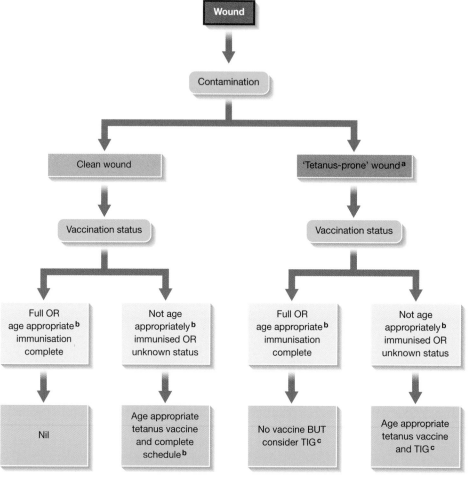

**Figure 39.1** Decision tree for use of vaccination and tetanus immunoglobulin (TIG) in wounds

a 'Tetanus-prone' wounds are described in Table 39.1
b For age-appropriate immunisation schedule see Table 39.2
c TIG, tetanus immunoglobulin

**Table 39.1** 'Tetanus-prone' wound

| | Any of the following factors indicates 'tetanus-prone' status |
|---|---|
| 1. | Contaminated with soil, faeces, saliva or foreign bodies |
| 2. | Associated with puncture, avulsion, burns, crush injury or compound fracture |
| 3. | Requiring delayed (>6 hours) surgical treatment, including burns |
| 4. | Patient experiencing systemic sepsis |

**Table 39.2** Age-appropriate immunisation schedule

| Age | Immunisation |
|---|---|
| 2 months | Primary dose 1 (DTaP/IPV/Hib/Hep B) |
| 3 months | Primary dose 2 (DTaP/IPV/Hib/Hep B) |
| 4 months | Primary dose 3 (DTaP/IPV/Hib/Hep B) |
| 4 to 5 years | Booster 1 (DTaP/IPV or dTaP/IPV) |
| 11 to 14 years | Booster 2 (Td/IPV, Td, Tdap or Tdap/IPV) |
| Adult | Booster within 10 years of last dose (Td/IPV, Td, Tdap or Tdap/IPV) |

**D**, high-dose diphtheria; **T**, tetanus toxoid; **aP**, high-dose acellular pertussis; **IPV**, inactivated polio vaccine; **Hib**, haemophilus influenza B; **Hep B**, hepatitis B; **d**, low-dose diphtheria; **ap**, low-dose acellular pertussis

*Minor Surgery at a Glance*, First Edition. Edited by Helen Mohan and Desmond Winter. © 2017 John Wiley & Sons, Ltd. Published 2017 by John Wiley & Sons, Ltd.

# What is tetanus?

Tetanus is an acute, life-threatening disease caused by the bacterium *Clostridium tetani*. It is characterised by rapid, progressive, severe muscular spasm and rigidity following wound contamination and anaerobic growth of *C. tetani*. It releases a potent neurotoxin, which causes synaptic blockade when taken up by nerves. As naturally acquired immunity does not occur, vaccination has an essential role in protection against tetanus. However, a decline in protection over time means that boosters every 10 years are required to maintain protection in the individual.

## Epidemiology

Any wound can be contaminated and sources of tetanus spores include soil, intestinal contents/faeces of humans and animals, such as cattle, sheep, horses, chicken, dogs, cats, rats and guinea pigs. The incubation period ranges from around 48 hours to several months, with most cases occurring within 14 days and individuals without full vaccination, such as young children and adults aged over 65 years, represent high-risk groups.

As a result of extensive vaccination programmes, World Health Organization (WHO) notifications have fallen by two-thirds to just 10 000 across almost a decade from 2002 to 2011, although WHO acknowledges significant under-reporting.

## The disease

Tetanus can present clinically in a local or generalised form.

Local tetanus is seen as muscle spasm restricted to the region surrounding the contaminated wound. It can last for several days to weeks and is associated with a low mortality, at approximately 1%, although it may progress to the more severe generalised tetanus.

Generalised tetanus is often recognised when spasm of the facial and neck muscles begins. Progressive involvement of the trunk and limbs is observed and spasm can last several minutes. When the spasm involves or affects the airway, as in laryngospasm or aspiration, tetanic airway compromise can be life threatening. Indeed, spasm can be violent enough to damage teeth and even fracture long bones. Additional autonomic nervous system effects can be seen as sweating, hypertension or arrhythmia. Effects can persist for several months, but generally improve after the first month. The mortality of generalised tetanus can be as high as 90% in high-risk groups, such as infants, the elderly and the unvaccinated, and so early recognition and management are crucial.

Diagnosis is made on clinical grounds, having ruled out alternative causes for observed muscle spasm, such as hypocalcaemia, phenothiazine toxicity and hysteria.

## Prophylaxis

The tetanus vaccine is a toxoid delivered as a cell-free inactivated toxin, adsorbed onto an aluminium adjuvant. Despite an efficacy approaching 100%, the protective effect may be inadequate beyond 10 years after vaccination.

The vaccine is administered as a 0.5 mL intramuscular injection, usually in the anterolateral thigh or deltoid.

## Routine primary (childhood) vaccination

The primary vaccination course should take place as part of a combined vaccination programme, as shown in Table 39.2. This offers protection against diphtheria, tetanus, pertussis, polio, haemophilus influenza B (Hib) and hepatitis B (Hep B). If interrupted, the primary schedule should be resumed, but not repeated, allowing one month between each remaining dose.

## Delayed primary vaccination

Unvaccinated adults and children aged 10 years or over should undergo a primary vaccination course of three doses, using tetanus vaccines containing low-dose diphtheria. Td/IPV is recommended, alternatives including Td, Tdap or Tdap/IPV (Table 39.2).

## Tetanus immunoglobulin (TIG)

TIG is used both in tetanus prophylaxis and treatment. It is not required for all wounds, but should be considered in 'tetanus-prone' wounds (Table 39.1). Decisions on tetanus prophylaxis should follow the decision tree shown in Figure 39.1.

When administered for prophylaxis, a single dose 250 IU (1 mL) TIG is given, usually intramuscularly. The dose is increased to 500 IU when: >24 hours have elapsed since injury; weight >90 kg; heavy contamination; or associated with infection or fracture.

For treatment of tetanus, the dose is titrated by weight, administering 150 IU/kg TIG at a number of different anatomical sites, intramuscularly or intravenously. High dose metronidazole and wound debridement are often required, along with anti-spasmodic pharmacotherapy. Admission to an intensive therapy unit is frequently required and regular reassessment should consider this necessity.

TIG is also recommended for 'tetanus-prone' wounds in immunocompromised patients, regardless of vaccination status.

### Further reading

Public Health England. *Immunisation Against Infectious Disease* (*The Green Book*), Chapter 30: Tetanus. London: Department of Health, 2013.

National Immunisation Office, Ireland. *Immunisation Guidelines for Ireland*. Chapter 21: Tetanus. Dublin, Ireland: Health Service Executive, 2013.

American Academy of Pediatrics. *Red Book: Report of the Committee on Infectious Diseases*, 29th edn. Illinois, USA: American Academy of Pediatrics, 2012.

# 40 Scalp lacerations

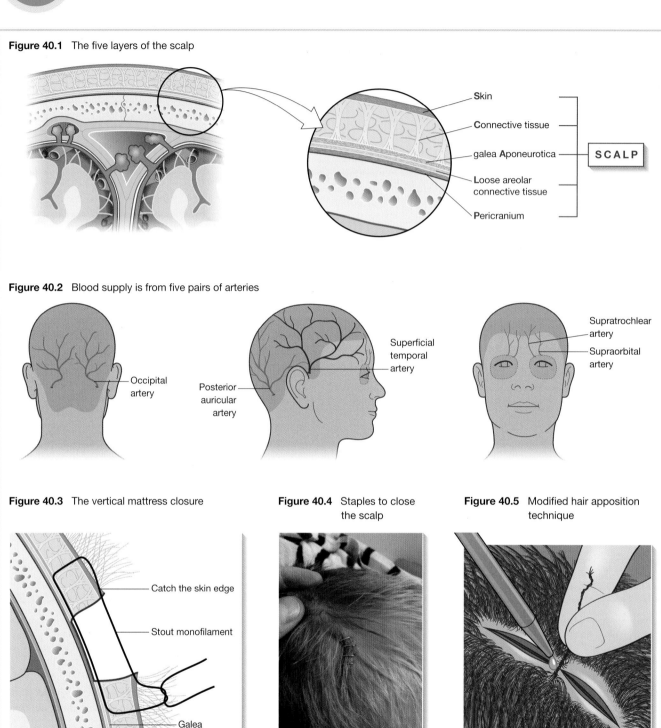

**Figure 40.1** The five layers of the scalp

Skin

Connective tissue

galea Aponeurotica

Loose areolar connective tissue

Pericranium

SCALP

**Figure 40.2** Blood supply is from five pairs of arteries

Occipital artery

Posterior auricular artery

Superficial temporal artery

Supratrochlear artery

Supraorbital artery

**Figure 40.3** The vertical mattress closure

Catch the skin edge

Stout monofilament

Galea

**Figure 40.4** Staples to close the scalp

**Figure 40.5** Modified hair apposition technique

*Minor Surgery at a Glance*, First Edition. Edited by Helen Mohan and Desmond Winter. © 2017 John Wiley & Sons, Ltd. Published 2017 by John Wiley & Sons, Ltd.

# Introduction

Scalp lacerations are a common consequence of minor cranial trauma; however, all patients should be managed using ATLS principles. The scalp is highly vascular and can bleed sufficiently to cause hypovolaemic shock and similarly the patient with associated serious head injury must not be missed.

Evaluation of the laceration should identify the cause of the injury and therefore potential for associated injuries, age of the wound, likelihood of contamination and foreign bodies. Examination should note the length, shape and depth of the wound, involvement of galea, or underlying bony defect and level of contamination.

CT brain imaging should be considered if there is visual or palpable evidence of skull fracture or if the patient fulfils 2014 NICE guidance (CG176). There are no indications for skull radiographs beyond the exclusion of radio-opaque foreign bodies.

One should confirm the tetanus status of the patient and, if appropriate, prophylaxis offered.

# Anatomy and neurovascular supply

The scalp has five layers (**S**kin, **C**onnective tissue, galea **A**poneurotica, **L**oose areolar connective tissue, **P**ericranium – mnemonic: SCALP) (Figure 40.1). The galea is a tough layer of fibrous tissue and its integrity or adequate repair is necessary for cosmesis, haemostasis and good skin edge apposition.

Blood supply (Figure 40.2) is from five pairs of arteries: three from the external carotid (occipital, posterior auricular and superficial temporal arteries) and two from the internal carotid (supratrochlear and supraorbital arteries). Because of the excellent blood flow to the scalp, wound infections are rare.

Scalp innervation is from C2 and all three branches of CN V can be remembered using the mnemonic: Z-GLASS (Zygomaticotemporal nerve, Greater occipital nerve, Lesser occipital nerve, Auriculotemporal nerve, Supratrochlear nerve and Supraorbital nerve).

# Wound preparation

Local analgesia (either plain lidocaine or lidocaine and epinephrine 1:200 000) should be given. Irrigation with 200 mL 0.9% normal saline is appropriate for clean wounds, and edges carefully debrided if necessary. Contaminated wounds should be cleansed with a mixture of 1:10 povidone-iodine solution and isotonic 0.9% normal saline. Hair trimming can be useful, but shaving is not a requirement unless it interferes with the mechanical aspects of closure. Hair is not contaminated with a high bacterial load, and once heavily soaked with standard wound preparation solutions, can often be flattened to either side of the wound with a comb.

Profuse bleeding can often be controlled with direct pressure for 15 minutes with or without local injection of lidocaine and epinephrine. If this fails, haemostatic control should be achieved with sutures rather than staples, ensuring circumferential closure of all layers of the scalp, for example, as shown in the vertical mattress closure demonstrated in Figure 40.3.

# Techniques of repair

## Suturing

This is the optimum technique in lacerations involving the galea. This is a key anchor for the frontalis muscle and so galeal lacerations >0.5 cm should be repaired separately with 3-0 or 4-0 interrupted absorbable sutures to prevent a cosmetic deformity. This also limits the risk of subgaleal infection. Thereafter, the skin should be closed with a second layer of 4-0 absorbable or non-absorbable interrupted sutures. Either horizontal mattress or simple interrupted suturing techniques are reasonable.

## Staples (Figure 40.4)

The quick application of staples makes them a good choice for the intoxicated or polytrauma patient. They are the optimum choice for lacerations involving the dermis, but without involvement of the galea, as they are non-circumferential and therefore limit tissue strangulation. The staples are applied approximately 0.5 cm apart. One should ensure good skin edge apposition, with slight eversion, using toothed forceps in the non-dominant hand.

## Modified hair apposition technique (Figure 40.5)

This technique is best for non-actively bleeding linear wounds that are less than 10 cm long, when scalp hair is longer than 1 cm. Five to fifteen opposing strands of hair either side of the wound are grasped with forceps or artery clips, and brought together with a simple twist. An assistant places one drop of tissue adhesive where the strands cross. This closure should be kept dry for 48 hours.

## Tissue adhesives

Appropriate as an alternative to 5-0 sutures in clean, non-haemorrhagic, well-opposed, superficial and small wounds only. The edges of the wound are closely opposed manually and the adhesive is applied to the wound edges with a gentle brushing technique. The edges are held opposed for 30 seconds before releasing. The repair is strengthened thereafter by applying more adhesive in an oval around the wound.

## Skin-closure strips

Although skin-closure strips can be effective for small, simple lacerations in low-tension areas with well-approximated edges, they are rarely appropriate in the scalp.

# Follow-up care

- Deep scalp lacerations may benefit from a pressure dressing for the first 24 hours, to prevent haematoma formation.
- Most scalp wounds, other than those caused by human or animal bites, do not require empiric antibiotics.
- Patients should be advised to keep the wound clean and dry using a protective dressing for at least 24 hours after closure and suture or staple removal should occur at the seventh post-operative day.

# When to refer

Scalp wounds with significant skin loss or extension onto the face warrant consultation with a plastic or maxillofacial surgeon. Neurosurgeons should be involved when potential penetration into the cranial vault has occurred.

# 41 Foreign bodies

**Figure 41.1** Fluoroscopic guided removal of foreign body (FB)

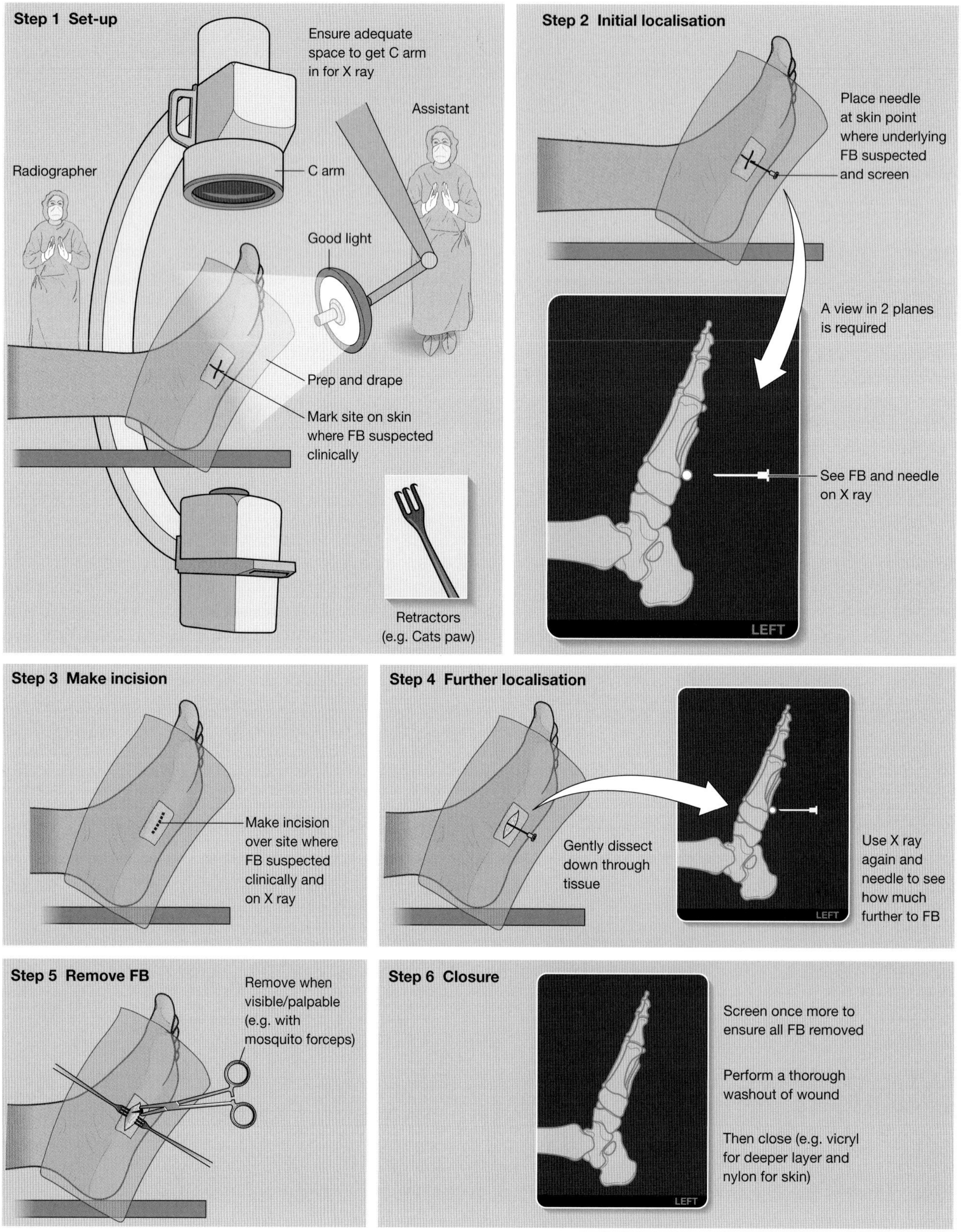

**Step 1 Set-up**

Ensure adequate space to get C arm in for X ray

Radiographer

Assistant

C arm

Good light

Prep and drape

Mark site on skin where FB suspected clinically

Retractors (e.g. Cats paw)

**Step 2 Initial localisation**

Place needle at skin point where underlying FB suspected and screen

A view in 2 planes is required

See FB and needle on X ray

LEFT

**Step 3 Make incision**

Make incision over site where FB suspected clinically and on X ray

**Step 4 Further localisation**

Gently dissect down through tissue

Use X ray again and needle to see how much further to FB

LEFT

**Step 5 Remove FB**

Remove when visible/palpable (e.g. with mosquito forceps)

**Step 6 Closure**

Screen once more to ensure all FB removed

Perform a thorough washout of wound

Then close (e.g. vicryl for deeper layer and nylon for skin)

LEFT

*Minor Surgery at a Glance*, First Edition. Edited by Helen Mohan and Desmond Winter. © 2017 John Wiley & Sons, Ltd. Published 2017 by John Wiley & Sons, Ltd.

# Introduction

This chapter pertains to foreign bodies resulting from a traumatic wound. Other sites common for foreign bodies include ears, eyes, oesophagus and airway. These are beyond the scope of this book.

Foreign bodies may be obvious on presentation, for example, if a nail is clearly protruding from a wound. Often, however, foreign bodies are not immediately evident on examination. A high index of suspicion is required in traumatic wounds and in patients with a history of a traumatic wound presenting later with infection.

# Assessment for foreign bodies

## History

History is important, and often provides the initial clue that there may be a foreign body.

Common sites for foreign bodies include the foot, hand and knee.

If it is a child, the parent or the child may report seeing a foreign body enter the wound, and may provide information as to what kind of object, e.g. shells playing on a beach, glass etc. The patient may complain of a sensation of something stuck in the wound or affected body part.

Try and ascertain what substance they think may be in the wound as it will provide a clue as to whether it is radio opaque or not, which is important in selecting an imaging modality.

Be careful to think of a foreign body in all traumatic wounds, as sometimes the history does not provide any clues at all.

Even if no history of a suspected foreign body is given, ask about exposure to glass etc.

As in all traumatic wounds, ask about tetanus status.

Remember, **DELAYED** presentation is common.

## Examination

Examine the wound carefully. Examine the surrounding skin. Sometimes a lump may be palpable consistent with a foreign body, but usually not.

Assess neurovascular status prior to administering any form of anaesthetic, and for evidence of tendon injury as in all traumatic wounds. To thoroughly examine the wound, some form of anaesthesia (local, regional block or GA) is needed followed by gentle but thorough washout of the wound and careful inspection.

Foreign bodies may be visible or may be occult. Avoid pushing a visible foreign body in further, rendering it more difficult to retrieve.

If no foreign body is detected and there is not a high index of suspicion of a FB, it is reasonable to close a wound in the emergency department after thorough irrigation and examination, and imaging where appropriate. Advise the patient that a retained FB is a risk and to represent if symptoms. Delayed presentation of a foreign body often occurs, with the patient representing with a wound infection, cellulitis or abscess. Always consider the possibility of a retained foreign body in patients presenting with a wound infection following a traumatic wound.

## Imaging

X-ray is the most common imaging modality utilised to locate a foreign body. This may be as an x-ray in the emergency department to locate if there is a foreign body, or to see the depth or extent of the foreign body. Fluoroscopy may be used in theatre to obtain serial views during removal of a foreign body. To see a foreign body on xray or fluoroscopy, it must be radioopaque. Even radio opaque items can be difficult to see if they are <2 mm. Ensure the patient is not pregnant prior to using ionising radiation.

Increasingly, ultrasound is used as a point of care investigation in the emergency department and can be applied to locate foreign bodies. There have been descriptions of ultrasound needle guided localisation of foreign bodies in the foot for example to reduce incision size (Nwaka et al). Radiolucent objects not seen on xray may be visible on ultrasound.

CT may be useful in preoperative planning of removal of large foreign bodies in stable patients, to assess whether vascular structures are at risk etc. CT or MRI are useful in locating foreign bodies not visible on ultrasound or xray.

# Removal of foreign bodies

**Consider:** Before attempting foreign body removal, consider if you have the appropriate setting, the appropriate expertise and access to the appropriate specialty. For example, a penetrating knife wound is not a simple foreign body and needs removal in theatre with appropriate blood products available and the appropriate surgical expertise and backup. Imaging may be needed to plan the surgical approach. Consider referral to orthopaedics if bone is involved, or to plastics if there is associated tendon injury.

If it is not possible to remove small or occult foreign bodies under direct vision, removal in theatre with image intensifier screening may be necessary. In children, removal in theatre under anaesthesia is usually necessary.

**Consent:** Counsel the patient that even if the foreign body is removed, it is difficult to exclude the possibility of other small fragments and to represent if still having symptoms. Occasionally, it may be prudent not to remove the foreign body if adjacent structures are at high risk, following an adequate explanation and discussion of options with the patient.

**Complete:** Minimise tissue trauma while retrieving a foreign body, use good lighting and positioning and retraction to maximise visualisation. Needle localisation may be used with image intensifier or ultrasound, to locate the foreign body and plan an incision site. Using a needle or artery forceps, place it over the site of the proposed skin incision and screen. If it looks to be in a good place on 2 views, then make your incision there and gently dissect down to reach the foreign body, using a needle to screen intermittently to aid localisation.

Confirm that the FB is gone with a post removal view in 2 planes on fluoroscopy if using it. Irrigate thoroughly prior to closure. Irrigate with NaCl 0.9% at high pressure.

### *Further reading*

Nwawka OK, Kabutey NK, Locke CM, Castro-Aragon I, Kim D. Ultrasound-guided needle localization to aid foreign body removal in pediatric patients. *J Foot Ankle Surg* 2014; 53(1): 67–70.

# 42 Facial trauma and lacerations

**Figure 42.1** Field block

A field block is a quick and effective way to numb an area being operated on

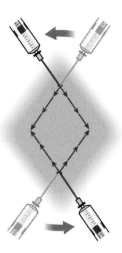

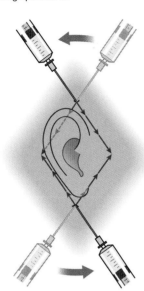

**(a)** This demonstrates how to perform a field block. A needle is inserted at two points and local anaesthetic is injected along the lines of the box, to numb the area within the box

**(b)** A field block is ideal when anaesthetising the ear

**Figure 42.2** Supraorbital nerve block and infraorbital nerve block

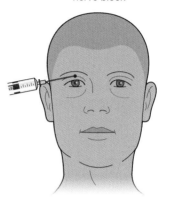

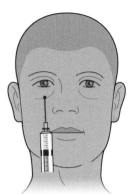

**(a)** The supraorbital nerve block is often used to accomplish regional anaesthesia of an area of the forehead above the eyebrow. The supraorbital nerve exits the skull through the supraorbital foramen, where it is palpable. It is often performed with a supratrochlear nerve block to achieve anaesthesia of a larger area of the forehead

**(b)** The infraorbital nerve block provides anaesthesia for the area between the lower eyelid and the upper lip

**Figure 42.3** Mental nerve block

The mental nerve is best accessed through the intraoral route

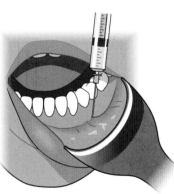

**(a)** The mental foramen is palpable. The cheek is retracted laterally. The needle is usually inserted between the 2 lower premolar teeth, towards the mental foramen

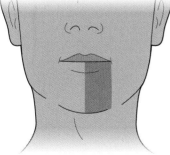

**(b)** This achieves anaesthesia of the ipsilateral lower lip

**Figure 42.4** Layered closure of the lip

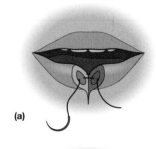

(a)

(b)

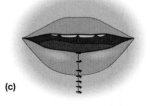

(c)

Aligning the orbicularis oris (a) will allow for accurate and easier placement of sutures in the mucosa (b) and skin (c)

**(d)** It is important to accurately approximate each of the layers of the lip

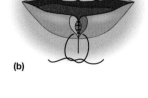

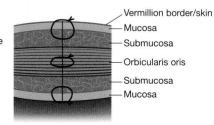

Vermillion border/skin
Mucosa
Submucosa
Orbicularis oris
Submucosa
Mucosa

*Minor Surgery at a Glance*, First Edition. Edited by Helen Mohan and Desmond Winter. © 2017 John Wiley & Sons, Ltd. Published 2017 by John Wiley & Sons, Ltd.

# Assessment of facial lacerations

Initial care of a patient with facial injuries should be guided by the standard trauma protocols with a standard primary survey. Considerations on primary survey in facial trauma include the following.

Facial injuries should alert the examiner to the possibility of airway compromise, cervical spine injuries, or central nervous system injuries. Management of the airway in maxillofacial trauma is always carried out with cervical spine control because up to 10% of facial trauma patients have cervical spinal injuries. Extreme caution should be exercised when attempting blind nasotracheal intubation; facial trauma is a relative contraindication with a potential risk of placing the tube intracranially in an obtunded patient.

Major haemorrhage can be managed temporarily with direct manual pressure. If cauterisation or surgical ligation is required, it is important to gain adequate exposure to avoid damage to adjacent structures. Active arterial bleeders can be tied off or suture ligated with a 4-0 vicryl suture. If direct visualisation is not possible because of excessive bleeding, apply pressure with sterile gauze, and take the patient to the operating room, so that adequate exposure is easier to achieve. Epistaxis is very common with maxillofacial injury. It can be controlled with packing. Obtain a nasal speculum and a bayonet forceps. Use either half-inch gauze soaked in antibiotic ointment or a nasal tampon. Half-inch gauze, soaked in adrenaline (1 : 200 000) is inserted into the nasal cavity. The tail of the gauze is left exposed and the gauze is layered along the floor of the nasal cavity by inserting the gauze posteriorly and then inferiorly until the roof of the cavity is reached. Commercially available nasal tampons are available. They are inserted into the nasal cavity, directed posteriorly, parallel to the floor of the nasal cavity. If the bleeding is posteriorly, occasionally a Foley catheter, with its balloon inflated will need to be inserted, this functions to reduce blood flow into the oropharynx and redirects it anteriorly, therefore requiring anterior packing too. When nasal packing is used, start the patient on prophylactic antibiotics to prevent streptococcal toxic shock syndrome and remove the packing as soon as possible. If bleeding is difficult to control, then radiological embolisation is usually effective.

## Central nervous system

Severe facial trauma is frequently associated with some form of traumatic brain injury. Most trauma patients with facial injuries undergo computed tomography (CT) imaging to rule out head and cervical spine injury.

### Secondary survey facial trauma

Evaluation for facial trauma requires examination of the following:

1 Skin and soft tissue
2 Bony structure
   - Clinical features that suggest fracture of the facial bones include: obvious deformity, pain, localised tenderness, palpable step, particularly in the malar region or zygoma
     - Signs of a basal skull fracture:
       i. Battle sign (bruised mastoid processes)
       ii. Haemotympanum
       iii. Racoon eyes (periorbital bruising)
       iv. CSF otorrhoea and CSF rhinorrhoea.
3 Eyes
   - 15–20% of patients with major facial trauma suffer vision-threatening injuries and there should be a low threshold for a formal ophthalmology review.
   - Inspection for subconjunctival haemorrhage, malposition of the eye or palpebral fissure, hyphaema – layering of blood in the inferior aspect of the anterior chamber. Requires urgent ophthalmology review due to the possibility of raised intraocular pressure.
   - Assess visual acuity and visual field, eye movements, pupil evaluation, optic nerve function and evaluation of the fundus.
   - Lacrimal apparatus: injury suggested by the presence of copious tears.
   - Pain, tenderness or palpable step overlying the orbital rim.
4 Nose and nasal passageway
   - Examine for evidence of septal deviation, septal haematoma or nasal discharge.
5 Ears
   - Inspection for haematoma
6 Oral cavity, dentition and occlusion
   - Intraoral lacerations
   - Dental malocclusion
   - Loose or fractured teeth
   - Mobility of the maxillary dental arch or dental alveolar segments.
7 Neurological assessment
   - Glasgow coma scale (GCS) assessment
     i. Motor response
     ii. Verbal response
     iii. Eye opening.
   - Full cranial nerve assessment
     i. Particularly trigeminal (V) and facial (VII) nerves
     ii. Trigeminal nerve: Sensory and motor components. Sensory branches to the face are the ophthalmic (V1), maxillary (V2) and mandibular (V3) nerves
     iii. Facial nerve. Sensory and motor components. Five major motor branches supply the muscles of facial expression: temporal branch, zygomatic branch, buccal branch, marginal mandibular branch and cervical branch.

## Documentation

Rough sketches of the patient's injuries should be recorded in the chart. Consent should be obtained to take photographs of the patient's injuries also. It is important to clearly document the findings during the examination. This is especially important for subsequent medico-legal reports. Remember that undocumented preoperative injuries may be attributed post-operatively to surgical intervention.

## Management of facial lacerations

Wounds should be cleaned as soon as possible, and to optimise the cosmetic result, they should ideally be closed within 24 hours of the injury. To allow for proper examination, adequate irrigation and repair of the wound, it must first be fully anaesthetised, for example, with 1% lidocaine with 1:200 000 adrenaline (± 8.4% sodium bicarbonate in a 9:1 ratio of anaesthetic:sodium bicarbonate) injected using a 25-gauge or 27-gauge needle. Injection of large volumes of local anaesthetic in the face will distort normal anatomy and make reconstruction very difficult. For this reason, it is preferable to use field blocks (Figure 42.1), regional nerve blocks (Figures 42.2 and 42.3) or general anaesthetic. Once fully anaesthetised, the wound is then cleaned thoroughly. This is achieved with a mild surgical soap and with the light use of a surgical scrub brush. Once the wound is macroscopically clean, it is further cleaned with copious amounts of normal saline.

All foreign debris must be removed. All dead, crushed and devitalised tissue must be debrided. Crushed tissue margins are debrided with a scalpel. The wound edges are freshened to help improve the final cosmetic result. Wound closure occurs once the wound has been adequately cleaned and debrided. The most important way to ensure the best scar is to accurately approximate the deep dermal layer.

The deep dermal layer suture is the most important part of closing a facial wound. A monofilament, absorbable suture is used to reduce the risk of infection. This suture will act to maintain sufficient tensile strength during the healing period. A common choice for the deep dermal stitch is poliglecaprone 25 (monocryl, Ethicon).

With a good, deep dermal suture, the function of the skin suture is to ensure more accurate approximation of the wound edges and to optimise eversion of the skin edges. This will further improve cosmetic outcome. The material used for the skin suture on the face is usually nylon or polypropylene (a 5-0 or 6-0) suture, usually placed as simple interrupted sutures. The non-absorbable sutures are usually removed at 5–7 days to reduce scarring.

An alternative suture for skin closure is a subcutaneous poliglecaprone 25 suture that can remain in place.

## Management of trauma to the ear

### Auricular haematoma

Inspect the ear for the presence of a haematoma. If present, this requires evacuation, using sterile technique, by making an incision over the overlying skin with a scalpel blade, or aspiration with an 18-gauge needle to prevent pressure on the auricular cartilage that can subsequently result in a reactive chondrogenesis.

Following drainage, a bolster dressing is applied to prevent re-accumulation of the haematoma.

### Ear laceration involving a cartilaginous defect

Irrigate the laceration thoroughly. Be conservative when debriding ear lacerations, to prevent cartilage exposure. Ensure that there is skin overlying all cartilage as this will help to prevent chondritis. A non-absorbable suture is used (6-0 nylon or polypropylene) to approximate the skin and perichondrium in a single bite.

The patient should apply topical antibiotic ointment twice daily and be prescribed prophylactic oral antibiotics for 5 days. They should be advised to return promptly if they develop a haematoma at the site.

## Management of eyebrow lacerations

Do not shave the eyebrow. Sterile technique, adequate irrigation and debridement should be performed.

Perform a layered closure. The deep layer should be closed with an absorbable suture (5-0 poliglecaprone or polyglactin 910). The skin should be closed with polypropylene (5-0 or 6-0). It is important to accurately align the brow elements when closing the skin.

## Management of lip lacerations

Management of lip lacerations requires accurate re-approximation of the injured structures, especially the vermillion–cutaneous junction, philtral columns and cupid's bow. These anatomic landmarks should be marked and aligned before injection with local anaesthetic that will result in distortion due to oedema following injection. A discrepancy in alignment of the vermillion border as little as 1 mm is noticeable at conversational distance. The vermillion border is re-approximated using a 6-0 nylon or polypropylene suture. The remainder of the skin is closed using a similar stitch.

Approximate each layer of a full thickness laceration, including the muscle layer (Figure 42.4). The orbicularis oris muscle must be re-approximated accurately using a 3-0 or 4-0 absorbable suture (poliglecaprone 25 or polyglactin 910).

The mucosa, including all of the surface of the lip, is closed with either 3-0 or 4-0 Polyglactin 910 (or chromic if available).

### *Further reading*

Sitzman TJ, Hanson SE, Alsheik NH, et al. Clinical criteria for obtaining maxillofacial computed tomographic scans in trauma patients. *Plastic and Reconstructive Surgery* 2011; 127: 1270–1278.

Gassner R, Tuli T, Hachl O, Rudisch A, Ulmer H. Cranio-maxillofacial trauma: a 10 year review of 9,543 cases with 21,067 injuries. *Journal of Cranio-maxillo-facial Surgery: Official Publication of the European Association for Cranio-maxillo-facial Surgery* 2003; 31: 51–61.

Shetty V, Dent DM, Glynn S, Brown KE. Psychosocial sequelae and correlates of orofacial injury. *Dental Clinics of North America* 2003; 47: 141–157, xi.

Hollier L Jr, Kelley P. Soft tissue and skeletal injuries of the face, in: Thorne CH, Aston SJ, Bartlett SP, Gurtner GC, Spear SL (eds) *Grabb and Smith's Plastic Surgery*, 6th edn. Philadelphia: Lippincott Williams & Wilkins, 2007.

# 43 Hand injuries

**Figure 43.1**  Examination of the flexor tendons of the hand

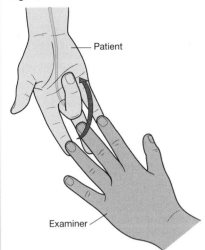

Patient

Examiner

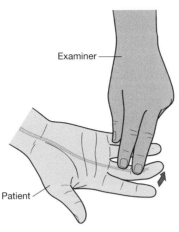

Examiner

Patient

**(a)**  Assessing flexor digitorum superficialis (FDS) function. The examiner should hold the fingers in extension, except the finger being tested. Ask the patient to flex the finger at the interphalangeal joint. If the patient cannot flex the finger, this suggests a cut FDS tendon.

**(b)**  Isolated testing of the flexor digitorum profundus (FDP) is performed by having the middle phalanx held in full extension by the examiner, and then asking the patient to actively flex the distal phalanx. Inability to actively flex the distal phalanx suggests that the FDP is cut.

**Figure 43.2**  Flexor zones of the hand

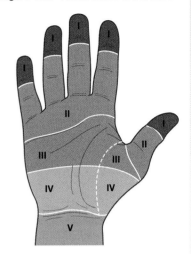

This is used to describe the level at which the injury has occurred as this has implications for tendon repair

**Figure 43.3**  Testing extensor tendons of the hand

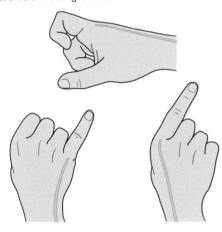

**Figure 43.4**  Extensor zones of the hand

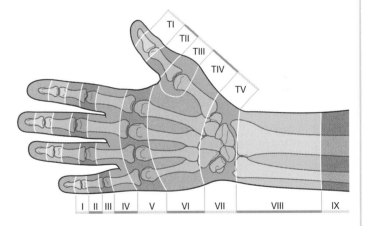

**Figure 43.5**  Testing the interossei muscles

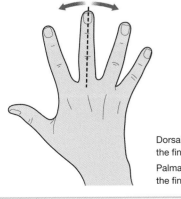

Dorsal interossei abduct the fingers

Palmar interossei adduct the fingers

**Figure 43.6**  Sensory nerve supply to the hand

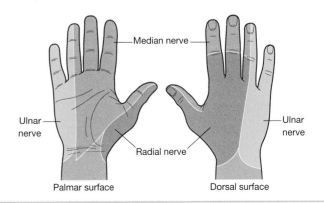

Median nerve

Ulnar nerve

Radial nerve

Ulnar nerve

Palmar surface

Dorsal surface

*Minor Surgery at a Glance*, First Edition. Edited by Helen Mohan and Desmond Winter. © 2017 John Wiley & Sons, Ltd. Published 2017 by John Wiley & Sons, Ltd.

# Assessment

Important features to ascertain in the history include age, hand dominance, occupation and hobbies, smoking history, when the injury occurred, mechanism of injury, pattern of symptoms and subjective functional deficit.

## Examination

Principle of hand examination is:

1 **Inspection:** Wound status (location, type, pattern), skin colour, scars, deformity, cascade, soft tissue loss

2 **Palpation:** Temperature, swelling, tenderness, deformity, pulses, sensation

3 **Motion assessment:** (Ensure the patient has adequate analgesia before assessing movement). Assess actively first and then passively. Record the active range of motion (AROM) and the passive range of motion (PROM) and note deficits present (Figures 43.1, 43.2, 43.3, 43.4 and 43.5).

4 **Stability assessment:** The examiner uses both hands, to hold both proximal and distal to the joint being tested. The examiner gently moves the joints passively to stress the ligaments that stabilise the joint. Assess for laxity at the joint that may indicate ligamentous injury.

5 **Nerve assessment:** Assess both sensory and motor function. The radial, median and ulnar nerves must be carefully examined for motor function (Figure 43.6).

Quick motor nerve tests:
- Radial nerve: Extension of the thumb
- Ulnar nerve: Get the patient to cross their fingers (interrosei muscle function)
- Median nerve: Recurrent branch: palmar abduction of the thumb, Anterior interosseous branch: making the 'OK sign' with thumb and index.

Sensory nerve tests: Examine the sensory distribution of the median, radial and ulnar nerves.

Digital nerves: Each digit has a radial and ulnar digital nerve. Reduced sensation on one border of the finger compared with an uninjured finger suggests digital nerve injury.

6 **Vascular assessment:** This relies on inspection (white discolouration with arterial insufficiency, blue and congested suggests venous insufficiency). A useful test is Allen's test to determine blood supply to the hand and to determine dominance and patency of the palmar arch.

To perform Allen's test:
i. Ask the patient to make a tight fist with their hand.
ii. You then apply occlusive pressure to the radial and ulnar arteries by compressing them at the wrist.
iii. Ask the patient to open their hand. Then slowly release the pressure on the ulnar artery. Observe the return of colour to the hand. This is an indication of ulnar artery patency. Normal return of colour is less than 5 seconds.
iv. Repeat steps (i) and (ii) again. Then release pressure from the radial artery to assess the patency of the radial artery to the hand. Again, this should be less than 5 seconds.

7 **Integument examination:** Examination of the skin, hair and nails.

# Management

## General principles in management of hand trauma

- Never blindly clamp a bleeding vessel as nerves are usually found in close proximity to the vessels.
- Arterial bleeding from a volar (palmar) digital laceration may indicate nerve injury (nerves in digits are superficial to arteries).

Suspicion of damage to a structure in the hand requires formal examination and repair in the operating theatre.

Table 43.1 Flexor tendon exam (Figures 43.1 and 43.2)

| Flexor tendons | | |
|---|---|---|
| **Tendon** | **Insertion** | **Function** |
| Flexor pollicis longus (FPL) | Base of distal phalanx of thumb | Flexion of the interphalangeal joint (IPJ) of the thumb |
| Flexor digitorum profundus (FDP) | Base of the distal phalanx D2-5 | Flexion at the distal IPJ (DIPJ) |
| Flexor digitorum superficialis (FDS) | Base of middle phalanx | Flexion at the proximal IPJ (PIPJ) |
| Flexor carpi ulnaris (FCU) | Pisiform and hamate | Flexion and abduction of the wrist |
| Flexor carpi radialis (FCR) | Base of the 2nd and 3rd metacarpals | Flexion and abduction of the wrist |

Table 43.2 Extensor tendon exam (Figures 43.3 and 43.4)

| Extensor tendons | | |
|---|---|---|
| **Tendon** | **Insertion** | **Function** |
| *Extensor compartment 1* | | |
| Abductor pollicis longus (APL) | Base of thumb metacarpal | Abduction of thumb at 90° to the palm |
| Extensor pollicis brevis (EPB) | Base of proximal phalanx of thumb | Abduction of thumb at 90° to the palm |
| *Extensor compartment 2* | | |
| Extensor carpi radialis longus (ECRL) | Base of 2nd metacarpal | Extension of wrist and radial deviation |
| Extensor carpi radialis brevis (ECRB) | Base of 3rd metacarpal | Extension of the wrist and radial deviation |
| *Extensor compartment 3* | | |
| Extensor pollicis longus (EPL) | Base of distal phalanx of thumb | Extension of the thumb |
| *Extensor compartment 4* | | |
| Extensor digitorum communis (EDC) | Base of middle and distal phalanges of D2-5 | Extension of the metacarpophalangeal joint (MCPJ), PIPJ and DIPJ of digits 2 -5 (D2-5) |
| Extensor indicis proprius (EIP) | Base of distal and middle phalanx D2 | Independent extension of the MCPJ, PIPJ, DIPJ of D2 |
| *Extensor compartment 5* | | |
| Extensor digiti minimi (EDM) | Base of distal and middle phalanx of D5 | Extension of the MCPJ, PIPJ and DIPJ of D5 |
| *Extensor compartment 6:* | | |
| Extensor carpi ulnaris (ECU) | Base of 5th metacarpal | Extension and ulnar deviation of the wrist |

If a hand surgery service is not available on-site, then it is best to liaise with a hand surgery centre early in the patient's management.

1 X-rays – ensure there is no bony abnormality or foreign body present. Two views are required (usually AP and lateral).

2 Keep the patient NPO.

3 Prophylactic antibiotics (usually broad-spectrum cover).

4 Tetanus prophylaxis.

5 Wound irrigation with normal saline and temporary dressing until formal procedure can be carried out.

Table 43.3 Intrinsic muscles of the hand

| Tendon | Insertion | Function |
|--------|-----------|----------|
| Abductor pollicis brevis (APB) | Base of the proximal phalanx of the thumb | Abduction of the thumb |
| Opponens pollicis (OP) | Radial side of metacarpal of the thumb | Opposes the thumb to the little finger |
| Flexor pollicis brevis (FPB) | Base of the proximal phalanx of thumb | Thumb flexion |
| Adductor pollicis (ADP) | Base of proximal phalanx of thumb | Adduction of the thumb towards the 2$^{nd}$ metacarpal |
| Lumbricals | Extensor mechanism | Flexion of the MCPJ and extension of the IPJ |
| Palmar interossei | Extensor expansions of D2-5 | Adduction of D2, D4 and D5 to the midline |
| Dorsal interossei | Extensor expansions of D2-5 | Abduction of D2-5 away from the midline |
| Abductor digit minimi (ADM) | Base of proximal phalanx of little finger | Abduction of D5 |
| Opponens digiti minimi (ODM) | Ulnar side of 5$^{th}$ metacarpal | Opposition of little finger to the thumb |
| Flexor digiti minimi (FDM) | Base of proximal phalanx of little finger | Flexion of D5 |

## Management of finger amputations

Never place an amputated digit directly on ice. The amputated digit should be wrapped in saline-soaked gauze and placed in bag. This bag should be placed in another bag of cold saline. Contact a local hand surgery service immediately to arrange urgent review.

### Digital nerves

Primary repair of a nerve is appropriate for injuries less than 2 weeks old if the injury is clean. Nerve repair will require magnification (loupes or microscope). An epineural repair of digital nerves is carried out using an 8-0 or 9-0 nylon suture with minimal tension. Post-operatively, the wound is dressed, the hand is elevated and the digit is immobilised. Peripheral nerves regenerate at 1 mm/day after the first 4 weeks as a result of Wallerian degeneration.

### Tendons

Most tendon lacerations require primary repair. As a general rule, flexor tendons are repaired with core suture (e.g. modified Kessler technique) with an epitendinous outer suture to provide extra strength to the repair. Extensor tendons can often be repaired in the emergency room. Approximation with a horizontal mattress suture (3-0 or 4-0 polydioxanone) is usually most appropriate.

### Vessels

Apply direct pressure and elevate the limb. Optimal repair of an injured vessel is within 6 hours, if required. It is important to remember that a vessel injury is often associated with a nerve injury, due to their proximity.

### Immobilisation

When applying an immobilisation cast, you have to protect your repair. For a flexor surface repair, a dorsal blocking splint is applied. For an extensor surface repair, a volar resting splint is applied.

When the hand needs to be immobilised, it should be in the 'safe position'. This decreases stiffness and allows rehabilitation. This involves:

1 Extension of the interphalageal joints
2 Flexion at the metacarpophalangeal joints to 60°
3 Wrist extension 10° less than maximal
4 Palmar abduction of the thumb

### Further reading

Berger RA, Weiss APC (eds). *Hand Surgery* (Volumes I & II). 1st edn. Philadelphia: Lippincott Williams & Wilkins, 2004.

Seiler JG (ed.). *Essentials of Hand Surgery. American Society for Surgery of the Hand*. Philadelphia: Lippincott Williams & Wilkins, 2002.

Thorne CH, Beasley RW, Aston SJ, et al. (eds). *Grabb and Smith's Plastic Surgery*. 6th edn. Philadelphia: Lippincott Williams and Wilkins, 2007.

## 44 Trauma assessment

**Figure 44.1** Primary survey

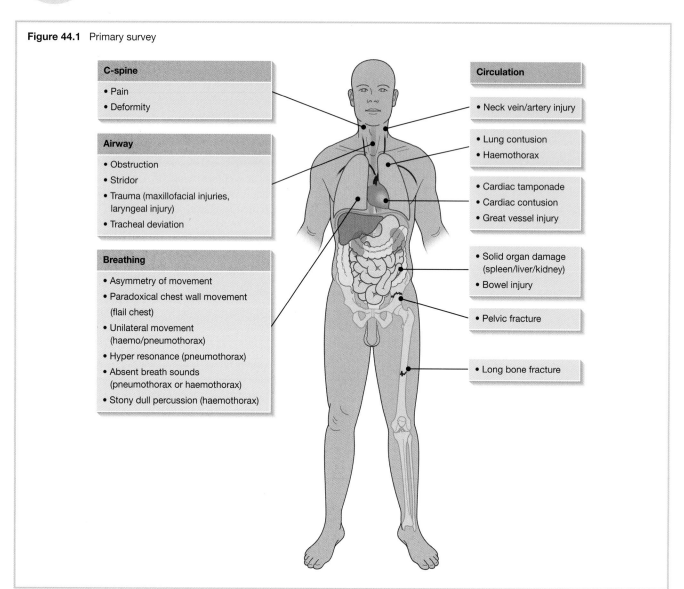

**C-spine**
- Pain
- Deformity

**Airway**
- Obstruction
- Stridor
- Trauma (maxillofacial injuries, laryngeal injury)
- Tracheal deviation

**Breathing**
- Asymmetry of movement
- Paradoxical chest wall movement (flail chest)
- Unilateral movement (haemo/pneumothorax)
- Hyper resonance (pneumothorax)
- Absent breath sounds (pneumothorax or haemothorax)
- Stony dull percussion (haemothorax)

**Circulation**
- Neck vein/artery injury
- Lung contusion
- Haemothorax
- Cardiac tamponade
- Cardiac contusion
- Great vessel injury
- Solid organ damage (spleen/liver/kidney)
- Bowel injury
- Pelvic fracture
- Long bone fracture

*Minor Surgery at a Glance*, First Edition. Edited by Helen Mohan and Desmond Winter. © 2017 John Wiley & Sons, Ltd. Published 2017 by John Wiley & Sons, Ltd.

## Mechanism of injury

Some of the scenarios where major traumatic injuries should be considered are as follows:

### Road traffic accidents

- Ejection from vehicle.
- Vehicle rollover.
- Steering wheel damage.
- Major damage into passenger area of vehicle.
- Vehicle versus pedestrian or bicycle.
- High speed vehicle crash (>30 km/h).
- Motorcycle crashes (separation of rider from bike).
- Fatality in same vehicle.

### Others

- Fall > 3 metres.
- Pregnancy.
- Age < 5 or > 55 years.
- Significant underlying medical conditions (heart or lung diabetes, bleeding disorder, anticoagulants, immunosuppressed).
- Significant assault.

    If any of these criteria are fulfilled, serious injury should be suspected.

## Primary survey

The role of the primary survey is to assess the patient for life threatening injuries. A systematic approach reduces the risk of missing a potentially fatal injury (Figure 44.1).

### Cervical spine

A cervical spine (C-spine) injury should be considered in all patients who have suffered a blunt trauma.

    Three-point neck stabilisation should be performed (hard collar, head supports and tape) until the C-spine can be fully evaluated.

    Non-radiographic clearance of the C-spine can only occur in a fully conscious, non-intoxicated patient with no barrier to communication between the treating doctor and the patient.

    In the presence of other injuries, C-spine clearance can be deferred until the patient can be safely evaluated.

    If radiological evaluation of the C-spine is needed, three views should be performed: cross-table lateral view (CTLV), anteroposterior view (AP) and an open mouth view to assess the otontoid process.

    It is essential to image the junction between C7 and T1. If plain films are inadequate, proceed to computed tomography (CT).

---

**Key point**

Rapidly assess level of consciousness, airway and breathing with simple questions such as:

- What is your name?
- Do you have any trouble breathing?
- Do you have any pain?
- Can you feel your toes?

---

### A Airway

Check for upper airway obstruction (clear by finger sweep or suction if necessary).

If patient unable to protect own airway:

- Chin lift to open airway
- Nasopharyngeal or oropharyngeal airway.
    Definitive airway:
- Endotracheal tube
    Surgical airway (facial trauma, disruption of upper airway, unable to intubate):
- Cricothyroidotomy.

### B Breathing

- Give supplemental oxygen.
- Assess respiratory rate.
- Look for symmetry of chest wall motion.
- Look for tracheal position (central or deviated).
- Monitor with pulse oximetry.

### C Circulation

➤ The most common cause of hypotension in trauma is bleeding.
- Assess pulse rate and blood pressure.
➤ Young patients may not show a drop in blood pressure until significant haemorrhage has occurred due to compensatory vasoconstriction and tachycardia.
- Achieve adequate venous access, two wide-bore intravenous cannulae,
- Commence warmed isotonic crystalloid infusion.
- Send blood for crossmatch, FBC, coagulation screen.
➤ In rapid haemorrhage, haemoglobin will not drop immediately and can be misleading.

### D Disability

Disability can be assessed by the AVPU scale:

- A – Alert, responds to voice appropriately, obeys commands
- V – Makes some response to voice
- P – Pain, responds to painful stimuli only
- U – Unresponsive to pain
- Capillary blood sugar and pupillary response should be included at this stage.
➤ A formal assessment of consciousness (Glasgow coma scale) can be performed later.

### E Exposure

- Fully expose patient to assess for bony injuries or sites of blood loss.

# 45 Psychosocial considerations

**Figure 45.1** Suspicious injuries for non-accidental injury

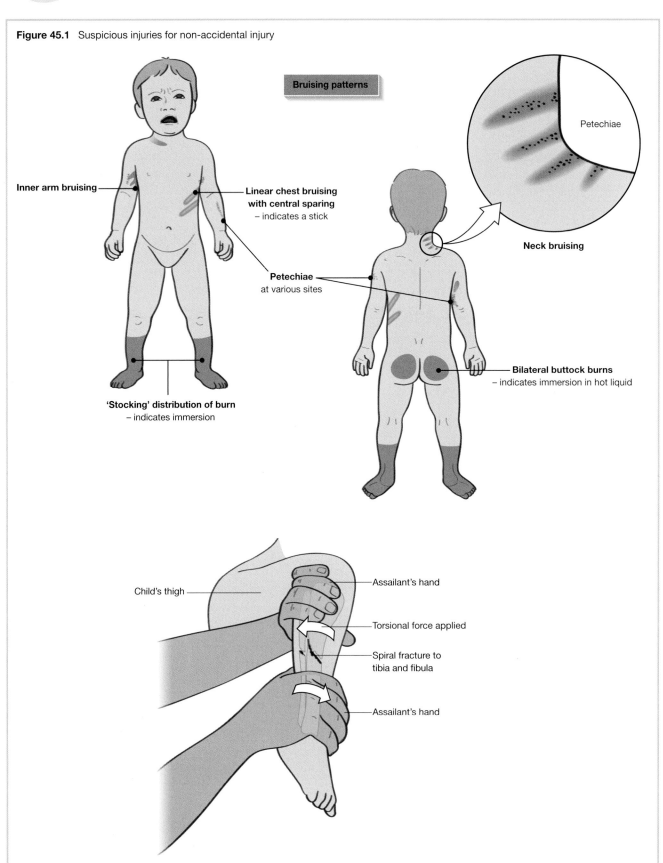

Bruising patterns

Petechiae

Inner arm bruising

Linear chest bruising with central sparing – indicates a stick

Neck bruising

Petechiae at various sites

'Stocking' distribution of burn – indicates immersion

Bilateral buttock burns – indicates immersion in hot liquid

Child's thigh

Assailant's hand

Torsional force applied

Spiral fracture to tibia and fibula

Assailant's hand

# Domestic violence

Domestic violence is injury or other abuse perpetrated by one person against another in a domestic environment.

Triggers to suspect domestic violence
- Multiple emergency department attendances with facial or axial injuries, frequently in the early mornings
- Attendance at a hospital outside normal catchment area
- Significant injuries sustained with a minor mechanism of injury (e.g. comminuted nasal bone fractures after a fall)
- Pattern injuries (blunt weapon such as a belt or stick)
- Defensive injuries – isolated ulna fractures, distal upper arm bruising, bruising to back or buttocks

Often, domestic violence victims hide the true cause of their injuries. It is important to establish an atmosphere of trust.

Patients with traumatic injuries should be seen in private. The privacy of minor procedures such as wound closure often present an opportunity for nervous patients to speak with their doctor in confidence. Other risk factors for domestic violence include: lower socioeconomic group, member of an ethnic minority grouping, alcohol / illicit drug misuse by either victim or perpetrator, pregnancy.

### Leading questions when asking about domestic violence
- *Do you feel safe at home?*
- *What happens when you and your partner disagree?*
- *Who else stays in your home? What other adults have access to your home?*
- *Do you think your children are ever scared at home?*
- *I notice you check with your partner before answering – are you worried you might say the wrong thing?*

## Dealing with domestic violence presentations

Involve senior staff early. Document carefully all aspects of the case in the medical notes. Offer the victim access to services that may help, such as emergency shelters, hospital and community social workers, and support groups for domestic violence. Encourage all victims of domestic violence to make a police report.

# Deliberate self-harm

Deliberate self-harm is self-poisoning or injury, irrespective of the apparent purpose of the act. However, the term is frequently used to describe those who self-harm without suicidal intent. While deliberate self-harm is not a suicide attempt, there is an increased long-term risk of suicide in those who self-harm.

Deliberate self-harm is associated with:
- Emotionally-unstable (borderline) personality disorder
- Prior child sexual or physical abuse
- Obsessive–compulsive disorder (OCD)
- Eating disorders

Deliberate self-harm has a strong female preponderance (4 :1). Many of those who self-harm go to lengths to disguise their injuries. Deliberate self-harm patients often say that self-harm relieves stress and allows some control over an intolerable situation.

## Typical patterns of deliberate self-harm
- Transverse incised wounds to inner aspects of forearms and thighs, using a razor blade, glass or knife
- 'Carving' – cutting words or symbols into skin
- Interference with healing of wounds (dermatillomania)
- Pulling out hair (trichotillomania)
- Overdoses

## Management
- Acknowledge that the wounds are self-inflicted
- Do not criticise or blame the person for self-harming
- Offer psychiatric or psychological help
- Close wounds with care, and give advice to avoid scarring. Self-harm scars can be stigmatising for life.

## Follow-up
- Arrange for all acute self-harm presentations to have a mental health assessment, ideally on the same day
- Ensure primary care is aware of the patient's presentation
- Patient with capacity *can* decline to see a psychiatrist, but need to be told the risks of doing so (5% risk of suicide within 9 years)

# Non-accidental injury in children

Non-accidental injury is any physical violence intentionally perpetrated by one person against another. However, the term is used primarily to describe physical violence against children.

## Key practice points

Childhood non-accidental injury is under-recognised and under-reported. Many countries have introduced mandatory reporting (with threat of legal sanction) for all healthcare staff. It is a complex area of practice with potentially huge consequences for both children and healthcare staff. **Involve senior staff early in all decisions.** Any child with a suspicion of non-accidental injury (Figure 45.1) should not leave hospital without review by a senior clinician and confirmation that the child is leaving to go to a place of safety. If there is any doubt as to the safety of a discharge, the child should be admitted to hospital, using an emergency care order if necessary, until child protection services have fully investigated.

## Triggers to suspect non-accidental injury in children
- Any unexplained, or poorly-explained injuries
- Significant injuries sustained with a minor mechanism of injury (e.g. femur fracture in a toddler with a simple fall)
- History changes with time, or between family members
- Injuries inconsistent with the developmental age of the child (e.g. tibia fracture in a 10 month old not yet walking)
- Delayed presentation for care (more than 24 hours)

### Burns
- Involving unusual locations (soles of feet, back, backs of hands, buttocks).
- Symmetrical burns.
- 'Glove and Sock' patterns.

### Bruising
- Involving unusual locations (medial arms, face, anterior neck, abdomen or groin).
- In particular patterns (parallel linear bruises indicate a stick, teeth marks, handprint).

### Further reading
When to suspect child maltreatment; NICE Clinical Guideline (July 2009)
Protecting children and young people: The responsibilities of all doctors; General Medical Council, 2012
Children First: National Guidance for the Protection and Welfare of Children. Government Press Office, Republic of Ireland (2011)

# 46 Incision and drainage of abscesses

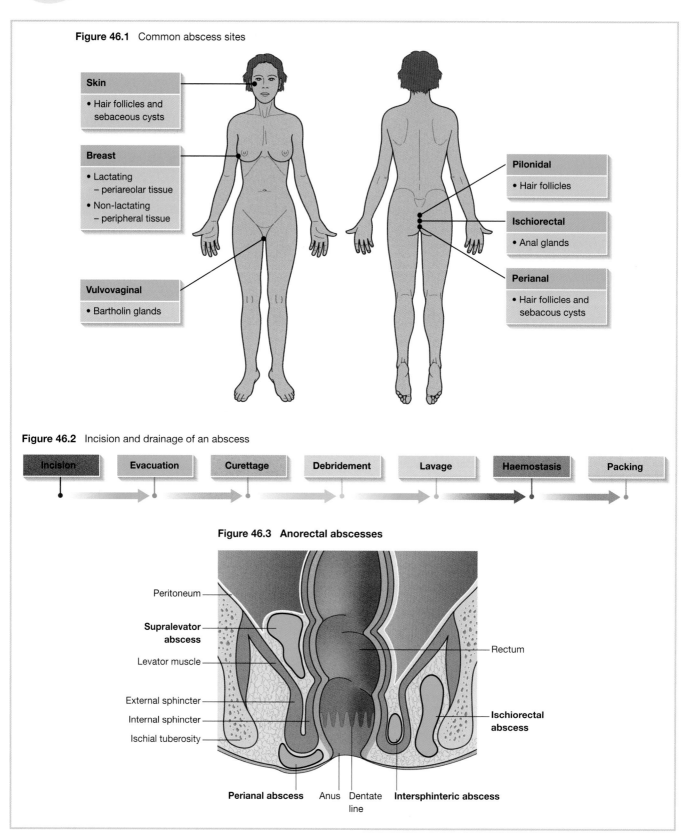

**Figure 46.1** Common abscess sites

**Skin**
- Hair follicles and sebaceous cysts

**Breast**
- Lactating
  – periareolar tissue
- Non-lactating
  – peripheral tissue

**Vulvovaginal**
- Bartholin glands

**Pilonidal**
- Hair follicles

**Ischiorectal**
- Anal glands

**Perianal**
- Hair follicles and sebacous cysts

**Figure 46.2** Incision and drainage of an abscess

Incision → Evacuation → Curettage → Debridement → Lavage → Haemostasis → Packing

**Figure 46.3** Anorectal abscesses

Peritoneum

**Supralevator abscess**

Levator muscle

External sphincter

Internal sphincter

Ischial tuberosity

Rectum

**Ischiorectal abscess**

**Perianal abscess**   Anus   Dentate line   **Intersphinteric abscess**

*Minor Surgery at a Glance*, First Edition. Edited by Helen Mohan and Desmond Winter. © 2017 John Wiley & Sons, Ltd. Published 2017 by John Wiley & Sons, Ltd.

# Definition of an abscess

An abscess is a localised collection of pus in a cavity. Abscesses occur as a result of the inflammatory response to pyogenic infections, in which the body walls-off the infectious material to prevent spread. Empyemas differ, with pus accumulating in a pre-existing cavity rather than a newly formed one. Abscesses may be superficial or deep. They do not always develop at the primary infection site but may occur distally, known as 'metastatic abscesses,' as a result of haematogenous, lymphatic or pyaemic spread.

# Causes

Most abscesses contain bacteria; only 5% are sterile. The microbiology and cause of localised abscesses relates to their anatomical location and often results from indigenous flora (Figure 46.1). Risk factors for abscess development include intravenous drug use, diabetes, immune-compromise, inflammatory bowel disease (anorectal abscesses), foreign bodies and surgical incisions.

# Clinical features

Classical signs of an abscess are:
- Rubor (redness)
- Tumour (swelling)
- Dolor (pain)
- Calor (heat)
- Function laesae (loss of function).

Systemic symptoms include swinging pyrexia, malaise and leucocytosis. Without treatment, abscesses have a tendency to track spontaneously to the nearest epithelial surface. External tracking is known as 'pointing' and results in the abscess discharging its contents. If the initial stimulus is expelled, the abscess may heal, otherwise a chronic abscess may develop with a sinus, intermittently swelling and discharging.

# Management

Simple rule: if pus is about, let it out! Superficial abscesses can be lanced under local anaesthetic, whilst those deeper to the skin need surgical drainage under general anaesthetic. Anorectal abscesses should always be managed under general anaesthetic to allow examination for underlying causes. Those within the body may require percutaneous drainage under radiological guidance or surgery.

## Aspiration

Frequently used to manage breast abscesses, this technique is only applicable if abscess contents are fluid. A large-bore needle is inserted under local anaesthetic and pus aspirated. Ultrasound guidance may be required and repeat procedures needed to treat the abscess.

## Incision and drainage (Figure 46.2)

Patients should be positioned to ensure adequate exposure (e.g. those with anorectal abscesses in the lithotomy position). Incisions should be made over the greatest point of fluctuance. It is important to be aware of the anatomy of the region involved to avoid important structures, for example, anal sphincters in anorectal abscesses, femoral vessels in groins. If there is any doubt regarding the relationship of an abscess to large vessels, a duplex scan should be performed prior to surgery to rule out pseudoaneurysm. The cavity interior should be explored and evacuated; a pus specimen should be sent for culture. The wall should be disrupted using curettage and necrotic tissue debrided. The cavity should then be thoroughly irrigated with physiological saline. Be sure to remove any foreign bodies that may act as a nidus for abscess formation. It is essential to ensure continued drainage of the cavity and therefore if necessary they should be de-roofed, using elliptical or cruciate incisions. This will encourage the cavity to heal via secondary intention, from the base by granulation, and packing with a non-absorbable ribbon material keeps the cavity open. It will need changing regularly until the cavity closes and so the initial incision needs to be large enough to accommodate this. These cases involve short hospital stays and the initial pack change – 24–48 hours post-surgery – may be carried out by ward staff or the district nurses, who will manage the wounds in the community. Surgical complications include pain, inadequate drainage, cellulitis, recurrence, and poor wound healing with scarring.

## Antibiotics

Given the impermeable nature of abscess walls to antibiotics, it is often difficult to treat abscesses adequately with antibiotics alone. They may prove beneficial in reducing inflammation, limiting further enlargement and sterilising the pus, creating a sterile abscess, an 'antibioma.' Antibiotics are not routinely required post-drainage unless there is persistent systemic or local infection.

# Anal abscesses

Most anorectal abscesses arise from infected anal glands, originating within the intersphincteric space. Tracking of the pus subsequently results in a variety of abscesses (Figure 46.3):
- Submucosal – these are very painful and occur within the anal canal, due to infections within the anal valves.
- Perianal – these are the commonest and are subcutaneous collections, typically arising from skin flora. The isolation of enterococci suggests an underlying communication with the bowel and warrants investigation.
- Ischiorectal – these develop within the ischiorectal fossa and are the most common location for horseshoe abscesses, in which pus tracks circumferentially around the anal canal.
- Supralevator – these are the rarest and form above the levator ani, usually as complications of intra-abdominal or pelvic infections.
- Intersphincteric – these are often over-looked as their deep location produces non-specific symptoms.

The abscess location determines its clinical presentation:
- Severe pain
- Rectal discharge or bleeding
- Superficial swelling and erythema (perianal/ischorectal)
- Palpable rectal/vaginal swelling (supralevator)
- Fever and inguinal lymphadenopathy.

Pain typically inhibits digital rectal examination and so rigid sigmoidoscopy should always be performed whilst under general anaesthetic to exclude further pathology. As a junior, you should never attempt to probe or lay open any sinuses or fistulae acutely; senior advice should be sought.

# Hidradenitis supparativa

A chronic skin condition characterised by infections of the apocrine sweat glands, it typically affects the axillae and groins. Disease spectrum ranges from single abscesses managed with incision and drainage to regional areas of skin with multiple chronic and recurring abscesses, interconnecting sinuses and scarring, requiring seton sutures or wide surgical excision and skin grafting. Long-term antibiotics may be used to induce remission and reduce flare-ups. Newer experimental approaches with biological therapy have been described. Consider dermatology referral for input.

# 47 Complications

## Background

Complications unfortunately occur in any type of surgery, and it is important to minimise the impact of complications on a patient's outcomes.

The key is to prevent them where possible, and to be prepared to deal with potential complications and manage them in a timely and professional manner.

- Prevent
  - Pay attention to timeout and human factors to ensure correct site surgery and avoidance of 'never events'.
  - Good set-up – ensure adequate lighting, equipment and systems to reduce error, for example, swab count, etc.
  - Meticulous surgical technique – achieve haemostasis, minimise tissue trauma.
  - Give clear post-operative instructions to nursing staff, the surgical team, the primary care team/GP and the patient themselves on aftercare.
- Prepare
  - Ensure your set-up is adequate to deal with major intraoperative complications.
  - Have a system in place to deal with post-operative complications.
  - Ensure the patient is prepared for possible complications by obtaining informed consent and giving the patient a follow-up plan. Make sure the patient knows what to look out for and who to contact if they experience complications when they are at home.
- Manage
  - Specific management varies depending on the complication.
  - REMEMBER CLEAR COMMUNICATION IS KEY.
  - The duty of candour is that medical professionals are obliged to openly disclose information about adverse events to patients.
  - The likelihood of medico-legal cases is much reduced if patients are communicated with clearly.

## Common complications in minor surgery

### Wound infection

Wound infection is a relatively common complication following minor procedures, with an incidence of up to 5%. Infection is usually due to colonisation of the wound from skin commensals. Wounds in the groins and natal cleft are particularly prone to infection.

#### Prevent

Perioperative measures can reduce the incidence of infective complications:

(a) Perioperative removal of skin hair
(b) Use of skin antiseptics (chlorhexidine/povidone-iodine)
(c) Meticulous haemostasis
(d) Use of prophylactic systemic antibiotics if indicated.

#### Prepare

Patients and caregivers should be told the signs of a wound infection and advised to seek medical attention if they are concerned.

- Superficial infection will present with swelling, erythema, pain and warmth around the wound.
- Deeper infection is associated with collection/abscess formation.

#### Management

- Superficial infection can be treated, following wound swab, with systemic antibiotic therapy and close observation of the wound to ensure resolution.
- Deeper infection requires removal of sutures, allowing the collection to drain. The wound should then be packed and allowed to heal by secondary intention.

## Seroma formation

A seroma is a sterile fluid collection that can accumulate in wounds, particularly following breast and inguinal surgery (inguinal lymph node excision biopsy). Seromas develop as a result of damaged tissue secreting fluid, leak of plasma from small calibre vessels and accumulation of lymph.

#### Prevent

Avoid excessive tissue dissection intraoperatively where possible.

#### Prepare

Seroma will present with swelling around the wound. Watch out for signs of superimposed infection.

#### Management

**Conservative:** seromas can be managed conservatively and observed.

**Aspiration:** seroma's can be aspirated under sterile conditions and a pressure dressing applied. Seromas can reform and may require repeated aspirations. In rare cases with repeated seroma formation, formal surgical excision may be required.

## Bleeding

Bleeding is a complication of any surgical procedure.

#### Prevent

Preoperatively enquire about bleeding diathesis and blood thinning medications. Follow local guidelines on cessation of blood thinning medications preoperatively. Intra operatively, take care to achieve haemostasis prior to finishing a procedure. Postoperatively, a pressure dressing may be useful if there is a slight ooze or a large cavity. If a cavity is very large, use of a drain may be considered.

#### Prepare

Watch out for signs of bleeding, including oozing of blood from the wound, haemodynamic compromise, or a haematoma.

#### Management

**Conservative:** Management of bleeding resulting from minor surgery usually consists of simple measures such as applying firm

*Minor Surgery at a Glance*, First Edition. Edited by Helen Mohan and Desmond Winter. © 2017 John Wiley & Sons, Ltd. Published 2017 by John Wiley & Sons, Ltd.

pressure over the wound and elevating the affected part, e.g. if bleeding from a wound on a limb. A pressure dressing may be useful.

**Surgical:** If bleeding persists, or haemodynamically compromised, urgent re-exploration in theatre may be necessary.

### Specific cases

Minor bleeding following haemorrhoid banding is common. Bleeding can occur immediately following banding, or seen at 7–10 days when the bands fall off. Conservative measures including reversal of anticoagulation and pressure, is often all that is required. Occasionally, it may be necessary to return a patient to theatre for control of the bleeding points.

## Haematoma

A haematoma is a collection of blood. Most commonly, haematomas present with bruising and swelling. Watch out for superimposed infection as blood provides an optimum culture medium for many organisms, for example, erythema, tenderness, systemic signs (e.g. pyrexia).

### Management

**Conservative:** If haemodynamically stable and the haematoma is small, it can be managed conservatively. Acutely, a pressure dressing may be applied.

**Surgical:** Tense haematomas should be drained – by reopening the skin closure sutures and washing out the wounds – and dressed, allowing for healing by secondary intention.

### Pitfalls

Patients can lose a lot of blood into soft tissue spaces. Patients who have a rapidly expanding haematoma and evidence of haemodynamic compromise may require blood transfusion and urgent re-exploration and packing in theatre, followed by attempts to isolate the bleeding vessel.

## Wound dehiscence

Wound dehiscence occurs when a wound closure fails and the wound 'breaks open'.

### Prevent

Wounds notorious for dehiscence include those in the pilonidal cleft, groin and over mobile joints. Risk factors for wound dehiscence include:

- Diabetes
- Obesity
- Long-term steroid usage
- Smoker
- Wound under tension
- Poor surgical technique.

Prevention of dehiscence requires a sound surgical technique. Skin edges should be adequately mobilised to reduce tension, with meticulous attention to haemostasis, use of appropriate suture material and square knot tying. Close monitoring of post-operative blood sugar in patients with diabetes, avoidance of heavy lifting and reduction in smoking can help prevent a dehiscence.

### Management

A dehisced wound should be washed out and necrotic or infected tissue should be debrided. In the absence of sepsis, a further attempt at delayed primary closure may be attempted; however, healing by secondary intention is the most likely outcome.

## Keloid scarring

Keloid scarring results from an overgrowth of granulation tissue within a wound. Keloid scars are composed of either type I or type III collagen. Keloid scars, which have the ability to grow beyond the limits of the original wound, may cause pain and are frequently disfiguring. Keloid scars developing over joints will result in disability.

### Prevent

Surgical trauma should be avoided if possible in susceptible patients. Patients at high risk are young patients and those with a history of keloid scarring. Areas at high risk are the neck and chest. Patients should be counselled preoperatively about the risk of keloid scarring.

### Management

Surgical excision of the scar is likely to result in further scarring. Keloid scars can be improved by a combination of corticosteroid injections, laser therapy, radiation therapy and cryosurgery. Consider referral to plastic surgery for advice. However, outcomes are often disappointing.

# 48 Difficult locations

## Where are difficult locations?

Locations that can be challenging include:
- Areas associated with poor blood supply and wound healing. The pretibial area is one example, as the skin is thin with a poor blood supply, and there is little subcutaneous tissue encountered before reaching underlying tendon.
- Cosmetically sensitive areas, for example, the nose, face or ear
- Areas where scarring can have serious functional consequences, such as the palmar surface of the hand.

Facial and hand injuries are dealt with in Chapter 42 and 44, respectively, and genital injuries are beyond the scope of this book; therefore, this chapter focuses on pretibial lacerations.

## Pretibial lacerations

Pretibial lacerations are common in elderly patients, particularly women. They often have very thin skin in this area, and the blood supply is poor with a tendon closely underlying the area. In addition, the skin is under tension. These injuries can lead to significant morbidity in patients who are often already compromised by co-morbidities.

### Assessment of pretibial lacerations

Pretibial lacerations may be superficial lacerations, or may be degloving-type extensive injuries.

#### History

Ask about mechanism of injury and consider other associated injuries. Ask about anticoagulation, as pretibial lacerations with accompanying haematoma caused by anticoagulation are a more difficult proposition than those not on anticoagulation. Ask about co-morbidities that may impair healing, for example diabetes mellitus, peripheral vascular disease and steroid use. Consider factors such as nutrition that may be optimised to aid healing.

#### Examination

Pretibial lacerations can be classified according to the Dunkin classification I–IV based on the degree of skin damage:
1. Dunkin I – simple pretibial laceration.
2. Dunkin II – pretibial laceration or flap with a small amount of skin edge necrosis or haematoma.
3. Dunkin III – pretibial laceration or flap with moderate to severe skin edge necrosis or haematoma.
4. Dunkin IV – pretibial degloving injury.

Always assess for evidence of peripheral vascular disease on examination – check pedal pulses, capillary refill etc. and document neurovascular status before focusing on the soft-tissue injury.

Assess whether the wound appears infected.

Consider other injuries and also the need for tetanus prevention. Specialist referral to plastics or vascular surgery may be required for some patients, for example in lacerations likely to need skin grafting, or in patients with diabetes mellitus or evidence of peripheral vascular disease.

## Conservative versus surgical

The first question in managing a pretibial laceration is not how to close the wound, but *should* you close this wound? The evidence supports early mobilisation to prevent further morbidity and taking a conservative approach using tape and dressings for simple pretibial lacerations. Dunkin et al. proposed a management algorithim based on their classification of pretibial lacerations.

| Management by Dunkin classification | |
|---|---|
| I | Clean (NaCl 0.9%), tension-free microporous dressings, e.g. Steri-strips®, supportive dressing, mobilise immediately |
| | Review day 7 and reapply supportive dressing |
| | Review day 14 – if not healing, manage as per Dunkin III with debridement and split skin graft (SSG) |
| II | Clean (NaCl 0.9%), debride non-viable skin and evacuate haematoma, tension-free microporous dressings, e.g. Steri-strips®, supportive dressing, mobilise immediately |
| | Review day 7 and reapply supportive dressing |
| | Review day 14 – if not healing, manage as per Dunkin III with debridement and split skin graft (SSG). If healing, continue current management |
| III | Clean (NaCl 0.9%), debride under LA, regional or GA, excise damaged skin and SSG, supportive dressing, mobilise immediately. Review day 7 and reapply supportive dressing |
| | Review day 14 – if not healing, debride and graft again as needed. If healing, continue current management |
| IV | Debridement and reconstruction under GA |

In patients on anticoagulants, correction of coagulopathy may be needed prior to debridement and grafting.

Remember, the remaining healthy skin should undergo minimal handling to avoid causing further damage.

## Infected pretibial lacerations

Always remember to consider infection in pretibial wounds and consider whether tetanus is needed.

For infected wounds, send a swab for microbiology, debride frequently to remove dead or infected tissue and use antibiotics for surrounding cellulitis. Review infected wounds daily.

### Further reading

Giele H, Cassell O. Chapter 13 Lower limb: Pretibial laceration, in *Plastic and Reconstructive Surgery*, pp 435–436. Oxford University Press.

Glass GE, Jain A, Pretibial lacerations: Experience from a lower limb trauma center and systematic review. *Journal of Plastic, Reconstructive & Aesthetic Surgery* 2014; 67(12): 1694–1702.

Dunkin CS, Elfleet D, Ling C, Brown TP. A step-by-step guide to classifying and managing pretibial injuries. *Journal of Wound Care* 2003; 12(3): 109–111.

# Index